Cervical Spinal Disorders

Springer
Singapore
Berlin
Heidelberg
New York
Barcelona
Hong Kong
London
Milan
Paris
Tokyo

Cervical Spinal Disorders

A TEXTBOOK FOR REHABILITATION SCIENCES STUDENTS

Editor

Sai Wing Lee

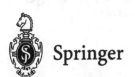

Springer

Sai Wing Lee
Department of Rehabilitation Sciences
The Hong Kong Polytechnic University
Hung Hom
Kowloon
Hong Kong

Library of Congress Cataloging-in-Publication Data

Cervical spinal disorders: a textbook for rehabilitation sciences students / editor,
Sai Wing Lee
    p. cm.
Includes bibliographical references.
ISBN 9814021296
    1. Cervical vertebrae--Diseases.   2. Cervical vertebrae—Wounds and
injuries.   3. Neck pain—Patients—Rehabilitation.   I. Lee, Sai Wing.
    [DNLM: 1. Cevical Vertebrae—injuries. 2. Spinal Diseases—rehabilitation.
WE 725 C4192 1999]
RD768.C44   1999
617.5'6--dc21   99-10460
DNLM/DLC   CIP
for Library of Congress

© Springer-Verlag Singapore Pte. Ltd. 1999
Printed in Singapore

Typesetting: Camera-ready by editor
SPIN 10717439   5 4 3 2 1 0

Preface

Neck pain is a disabling disease, which can decrease our work performance, disturb our lifestyle and limit our social activities. As patients with neck problems are frequently referred for physiotherapy and/or occupational therapy, a comprehensive understanding of the cervical spine and its pathologies is important for both physiotherapists and occupational therapists. Therefore, the aim of this textbook is to provide rehabilitation science students a framework to study in this field. It is hoped that the content of this text can assist them to integrate the knowledge of different areas related to the cervical spine. It is also hoped that students can appreciate the role of different professionals in treating patients with cervical spinal disorders.

Sai Wing Lee

Contents

Part I. Fundamentals of cervical spinal disorders

1. Anatomy of the cervical spine and its clinical implications 3
   William W.N. Tsang
2. Essences of neurovascular systems of the cervical spine 17
   Margaret Kit Yi Mak
3. Biomechanics of the cervical spine 33
   Sai Wing Lee

Part II. Cervical spinal disorders in clinical practice

4. Common conditions of the cervical spine 49
   Sai Wing Lee
5. Clinical investigations of cervical spinal disorders 63
   Raymond Ping Hong Chin
6. Diagnostic imaging of the cervical spine 77
   James F. Griffith
7. Cervical spinal trauma and its surgical treatment 95
   Y.L. Lee
8. Orthoses for cervical spinal disorders 103
   M.S. Wong

Part III. Occupational and sports injuries of the neck

9. Occupational disorders of the neck 119
   Bosco Tak Wai Chan
10. Ergonomics of the shoulder and neck 135
    Simon S. Yeung
11. Sports injuries of the cervical spine 147
    Candy Wu

Part IV. Rehabilitation of patients with cervical spinal disorders

12. Principles of neck pain rehabilitation   161
    Thomas T.W. Chiu
13. Electrotherapy for cervical spinal disorders   173
    Grace P.Y. Szeto
14. Exercise therapy for cervical spinal disorders   193
    Herman M.C.Lau
15. Manual therapy for cervical spinal disorders   209
    Ella W. Yeung
16. Vocational rehabilitation of patients with cervical spinal   227
    disorders
    Cecilia W.P. Tsang-Li
17. Community education on neck care   239
    Hon Sun Lai

Part V. Advanced studies in cervical spinal disorders

18. Current research in neck pain and its rehabilitation   253
    Sai Wing Lee
19. Outcome assessment of neck pain rehabilitation   263
    Lawrence C.W. Fung

Contributors

William W.N. Tsang, PDPT(HKPU), MPhil (CUHK)
Assistant Professor, The Department of Rehabilitation Sciences, The Hong Kong Polytechnic University, Hong Kong (SAR), China.

Margaret Kit Yi Mak, PDPT(HKPU), MAppSc(Curtin)
Assistant Professor, The Department of Rehabilitation Sciences, The Hong Kong Polytechnic University, Hong Kong (SAR), China.

Sai Wing Lee, MSc(Surr), PhD(Lond)
Assistant Professor, The Department of Rehabilitation Sciences, The Hong Kong Polytechnic University, Hong Kong (SAR), China.

Raymond Ping Hong Chin, FRCS, FHKAM
Senior Medical Officer, Department of Orthopaedic & Traumatology, The Queen Elizabeth Hospital, Hong Kong (SAR), China.

James F. Griffith, MRCP, FRCR
Associate Professor, Department of Diagnostic Radiology & Organ Imaging, The Prince of Wales Hospital, Shatin, Hong Kong (SAR), China.

Yuen Lun Lee, MBBS(HKU), FHKAM(Orthop)
Adjunct Assistant Professor, Department of Orthopaedic & Traumatology, The Prince of Wales Hospital, Shatin, Hong Kong (SAR), China.

Man Sang Wong, CPO(HK), MPhil(HKPU)
Assistant Professor, Jockey Club Rehabilitation Engineering Centre, The Hong Kong Polytechnic University, Hong Kong (SAR), China.

Bosco Tak Wai Chan, PDPT(HKPU), MScSp(UNSW)
Physiotherapist,The RehabAid, The Hong Kong Polytechnic University, Hong Kong (SAR), China.

Simon S. Yeung, PDPT(HKPU), MPhil(CUHK)
Assistant Professor, The Department of Rehabilitation Sciences, The Hong Kong Polytechnic University, Hong Kong (SAR), China.

Candy Wu, BAppSc(PT)
Sport Physiotherapists in Charge, Sport Medicine Department, The Hong Kong Sport Institute, Shatin, Hong Kong (SAR), China.

Thomas T. W. Chiu, PRCert (Spinal Manip), MPhtySt (UQ)
Assistant Professor, The Department of Rehabilitation Sciences, The Hong Kong Polytechnic University, Hong Kong (SAR), China.

Grace P.Y. Szeto, BSc(PT)(TU), MAppSc(Curtin)
Assistant Professor, The Department of Rehabilitation Sciences, The Hong Kong Polytechnic University, Hong Kong (SAR), China.

Herman M.C. Lau, PDPT(HKPU), GradDipManipPhysio(Syd)
Department Manager,The Physiotherapy Department, The Prince of Wales Hospital, Shatin, Hong Kong (SAR), China.

Ella W. Yeung, BSc(PT)(South Aust), MSc(PT)(South Aust)
Assistant Professor, The Department of Rehabilitation Sciences, The Hong Kong Polytechnic University, Hong Kong (SAR), China.

Cecilia W.P. Tsang-Li, PDOT(HUPU), MPhil(CUHK)
Associate Professor, The Department of Rehabilitation Sciences, The Hong Kong Polytechnic University, Hong Kong (SAR), China.

Hon Sun Lai, BSc(Murd), MAppSc(Curtin)
Physiotherapy Clinic Manager, The Department of Rehabilitation Sciences, The Hong Kong Polytechnic University, Hong Kong (SAR), China.

Lawrence C.W. Fung, MSc(Healthcare)(HKPU)
Department Manager, The Physiotherapy Department, The Kwong Wah Hospital, Hong Kong (SAR), China.

PART I

Fundamentals of Cervical Spinal Disorders

CHAPTER 1

ANATOMY OF THE CERVICAL SPINE AND ITS CLINICAL IMPLICATIONS

William W.N. Tsang

INTRODUCTION

The spine consists of 33 vertebrae and is divided into five separate regions. They are the cervical, thoracic, lumbar, sacral and coccygeal regions.

Although vertebrae show regional differences, they share a common structural pattern. A typical vertebra is comprised of a vertebral body and a vertebral arch (Figures 1a and 1b). The vertebral body is the anterior part of the vertebra, which is large and heavy. Its function is to support the body weight.

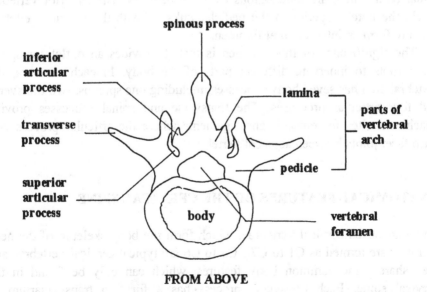

FROM ABOVE

Figure 1a. Overtop view of a typical vertebra (the second lumbar vertebra).

2

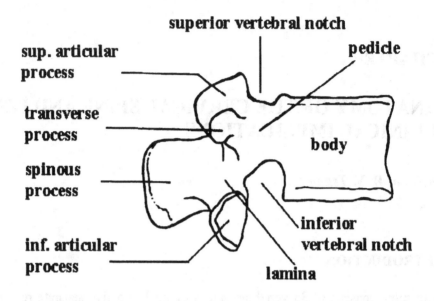

Figure 1b. Side view of a typical vertebra (the second lumbar vertebra).

The vertebral arch consists of a pair of pedicles, which form the sides of the arch, and a pair of flattened laminae, which complete the arch posteriorly. The vertebral arch encloses the vertebral foramen, providing a passage for the spinal cord. There are indentations over the pedicles. The superior vertebral notch, the notch superior to the pedicle, links up with the inferior vertebral notch to form an intervertebral foramen.

The significance of this foramen is that it provides an outlet for spinal nerve roots to innervate different parts of the body. In each vertebra, the vertebral arch has seven bony processes, including one spinous, two transverse and four articular processes. The transverse and spinal processes provide attachment sites for muscles and ligaments where the articular process will form facet joints between adjacent vertebrae.

ANATOMICAL FEATURES OF THE CERVICAL SPINE

There are seven cervical vertebrae, which form the bony skeleton of the neck and they are termed as C1 to C7. C3 to C6 are typical cervical vertebrae and they share some common bony features, which can only be found in the cervical spine. Each transverse process has a foramen transversarium or foramen of the transverse process. Vertebral arteries will then pass through these foraminae transversarium to supply blood to the brain, with the exception of C7. The spinous processes of these typical vertebrae are small and bifid shaped. The vertebral bodies are relatively small and their lateral dimensions are broader than the antero-posterior dimensions. The vertebral foramen is large and triangular in shape. The articular facets of the superior articular processes are small and flat. All these articular facets face superiorly and posteriorly.

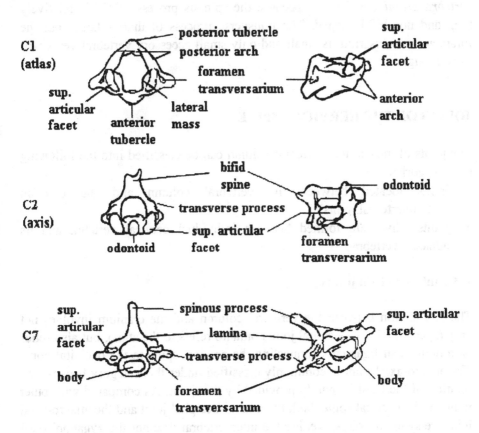

Figure 2. Cervical vertebrae of C1, C2, and C7.

C1, C2 and C7 are atypical cervical vertebrae (Figure 2). C1 (atlas) consists of a pair of strong lateral masses, which are linked anteriorly by anterior arch and posteriorly by posterior arch. On each side, the lateral mass possesses a superior articular facet, which articulates with the occipital condyle of the skull bone. Below, the inferior articular facet articulates with C2. The transverse process of atlas is palpable between the mastoid process and the mandibular angle. The anterior arch of the atlas has a small anterior tubercle in the midline. The inner surface of the anterior arch articulates with the dens of

C2. Posteriorly, in the place of a true spinous process, the atlas has a midline posterior tubercle where the two halves posterior arches meet. C2 (axis) has a peg-like odontoid process (dens). The axis is unique because the odontoid process can be fitted into the space left by the "missing" body of atlas. The odontoid process has an articular facet, which can articulate with the anterior arch of atlas. It is then held in position by a transverse ligament of the atlas, which can limit the horizontal displacement of the atlas. C7 is known as *vertebra prominens*. This is because the spinous process of C7 is relatively long and non-bifid shaped. The transverse process of that is large, but the foramen transversarium is small and only small accessory vertebral veins will pass through.

JOINTS OF THE CERVICAL SPINE

The joints of the cervical vertebral column can be classified into the following two categories:
- joints located between the vertebral column and the cranium (craniovertebral joints)
- joints which are formed between individual cervical vertebra and its adjacent vertebrae

1. Craniovertebral joints

The articulation between the vertebral column and the cranium involves not only a pair of atlanto-occipital joints (atlanto refers to the atlas), but also relies on a number of ligaments connecting the cervical spine to the occipital bone. The atlanto-axial joint is commonly classified under this category because the rotation of the head is mainly provided by this joint. As compared with other joints of the cervical spine, both the atlanto-occipital joint and the atlanto-axial joint are synovial joints. Neither the intervertebral disc nor the zygapophyseal (facet) joints are present between C1 and C2 vertebrae.

1.1   Atlanto-occipital joint

The atlanto-occipital joint is an ellipsoid joint. The superior articular facet of the lateral mass of the atlas articulates with the condyles of occipital bone. Each joint has a thin but loose articular capsule. The capsule is lined with synovial membrane on the inside and reinforced by anterior and posterior atlanto-occipital membranes, which connect the skull and C1 (Figure 3). The anterior atlanto-occipital membrane is a broad and dense band. It passes between the anterior margin of foramen magnum at the skull base and the upper border of the anterior arch of the atlas. The anterior atlanto-occipital membrane is further strengthened by the continuation of anterior longitudinal ligament in the anterior side of the cervical spine. The posterior atlanto-occipital membrane is a broad but thin band. It begins from the posterior margin of the foramen magnum and ends at the upper border of the posterior arch of the atlas. On each side, the membrane arches over the groove of the vertebral artery, making an opening for the C1 spinal nerve to communicate with body parts outside the spine.

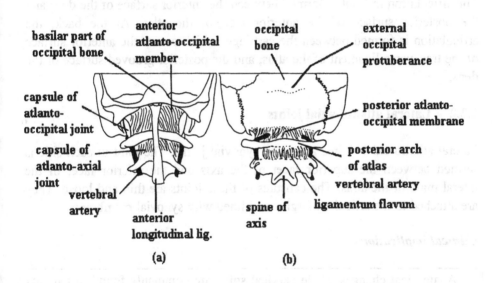

(a)   (b)

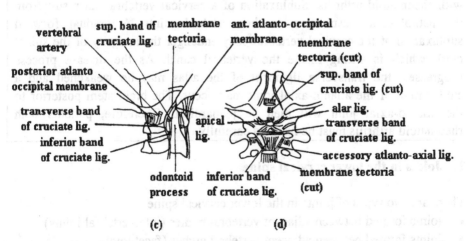

(c)   (d)

Figure 3. Atlanto-occipitial joints: (a) anterior view; (b) posterior view; (c) sagittal view; (d) coronal view.

1.2   Atlanto-axial joint (C1/2)

The atlanto-axial joint comprises three joints, including a median atlanto-axial joint and two lateral atlanto-axial joints.

1.2.1   Median atlanto-axial joint

This joint is a pivot synovial joint formed by the dens of C2 and a ring shaped structure of C1 composed of the anterior arch of the atlas and the transverse ligament. There are two articulation surfaces in the median atlanto-axial joint. The articulation in front is formed between the anterior surface of the dens and the posterior surface of the anterior arch of the atlas. At the back, the articulation is formed between the cartilage, which covers the anterior surface of the transverse ligament of the atlas, and the posterior grooved surface of the dens.

1.2.2   Lateral atlanto-axial joints

Lateral atlanto-axial joints are plane synovial joints. The joint in each side is formed between the superior facet of the axis and the inferior facet of the lateral mass of the atlas. The capsules of these joints are thin and loose. They are attached to the articular margins and lined with synovial membrane.

Clinical implications

Anatomical changes of the cervical spine are commonly found in patients with rheumatoid arthritis. Subluxation of a cervical vertebra can result from the pathological destruction of the vertebral joints. A gradual forward subluxation of the cervical vertebrae may endanger the integrity of the spinal cord, which is sitting inside the vertebral canal. As the disease process progresses, the transverse ligament of the atlas may be weakened and a subluxation of the atlanto-axial joint may occur. The brain stem posterior to the atlanto-axial joint will then be jeopardised. Therefore, patients with rheumatoid arthritis must be handled carefully.

2.   Joints in the lower cervical spine

There are two types of joints in the lower cervical spine:
• joints formed between adjacent vertebral bodies (intervertebral joints)
• joints formed between adjacent vertebral arches (facet joints)

2.1 Intervertebral joint

Intervertebral joint is symphysis joint formed between a pair of adjacent cervical vertebrae. The articular surfaces involve both the upper and lower surfaces of vertebral bodies. These surfaces are covered by thin layers of hyaline cartilage with an intervertebral disc sandwiched in between. The vertebral bodies are externally stabilised by the anterior and posterior longitudinal ligaments (Figure 4). Both ligaments firmly adhere to the intervertebral disc and the margin of the vertebral bodies. Excessive movements of the cervical spine can then be prevented.

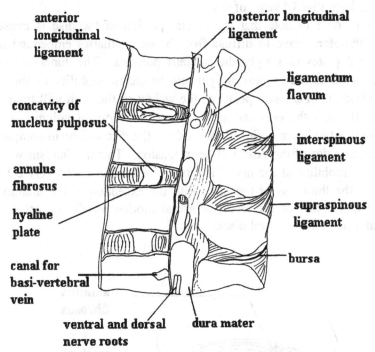

Figure 4. Median section of an intervertebral disc and its associated ligaments.

Intervertebral disc

Intervertebral discs are made of fibrocartilage and constitute 20 to 30% of the vertebral column height, excluding the first two cervical vertebrae. The shape and thickness of the disc vary from level to level. For example, the intervertebral discs are relatively thick in the anterior side in the cervical and lumbar regions. This contributes to the anterior convexity of the spinal alignment in both these regions. Each disc consists of a peripheral and a central portion (Figure 5). The peripheral portion is termed *annulus fibrosus*, which is made up of fibrocartilage. The collagen fibres are arranged in a concentric lamellae pattern and aligned obliquely in relation to the adjacent vertebral bodies. However, their inclination is reversed in alternate lamellae. The central portion is termed *nucleus pulposus* and it contains pulpy tissue mass. It is composed of a very loose and translucent network of fine fibrous strands that lie in a mucoprotein gel. The nucleus pulposus generally lies near the posterior boarder of the disc. The peripheral part of the disc is nourished by the extrinsic arterial system of the cervical spine. The water content of the nucleus pulposus ranges from 70 to 90% in normal adults. However, it will decrease with age and the soft gelatinous material will be gradually replaced by fibrocartilage after 10 years of age.

It is important to note that the central portion of the disc is avascular. Nutrients, therefore, have to diffuse from blood capillaries embedded in the vertebral end plates to supply the nucleus pulposus. The functions of the intervertebral discs are to bear weight and to enable mobility of the spine. When the body is in an erect position, the weight of the skull will transmit to the thorax through the cervical spine. When the vertebral column is either flexed, extended or laterally flexed, one side of the disc will be in compression whereas other sides of the disc will be in tension. This mechanism will then facilitate the mobility of the neck. The range of motion of the cervical spine depends on the thickness of the disc, with the exception of the atlanto-axial joint. The major part of the range of spinal motion usually occurs at those levels with thick intervertebral discs.

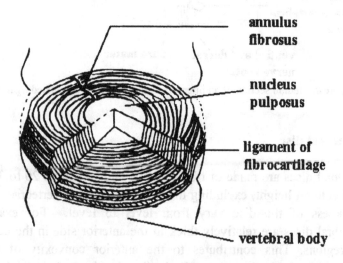

annulus fibrosus

nucleus pulposus

ligament of fibrocartilage

vertebral body

Figure 5. Main structural features of an intervertebral disc.

Clinical implications

Prolapsed intervertebral disc is commonly caused by wear and tear of the annulus fibrosus. Protrusion of the nucleus pulposus usually occurs posterolaterally, where the annulus fibrosus is weak and poorly supported by the posterior longitudinal ligament. The discs between C5-C6 and C6-C7 are the most frequently affected levels. It is believed that a small cervical disc protrusion may irritate pain sensitive receptors in the posterior longitudinal ligament, causing neck pain. However, if the size of the protrusion lump is large, it may compress upon spinal nerve roots or even the spinal cord immediately next to the disc, leading to neurological deficit. Fortunately, the incidence rate of prolapsed cervical disc is less common than lumbar disc protrusion in clinical practice.

2.2   Facet joints

The joints of the vertebral arches (zygapophyseal or facet joints) are synovial plane joints. The articular surfaces comprise the superior and inferior facets of the articular processes of a pair of adjacent vertebral segments. The articular facets are covered with hyaline cartilage. The articular capsule is thin and loose and attaches just peripheral to the articular facets margins.

Clinical implications

Since the facet joints of the cervical spine are in close proximity to the cervical spinal nerves, the nerves are relatively easily trapped at the intervertebral foramina, in the case of trauma or osteophytes encroachment.

LIGAMENTS OF THE CERVICAL SPINE

Ligaments connecting the axis and cranium are illustrated in Figure 3. The ligaments that directly connect the axis and cranium are membrana tectoria, alar ligaments and apical ligaments.

- The membrana tectoria is a strong and broad ligamentous band situated inside the vertebral canal. It covers the basilar part of the occipital bone, the posterior surface of the body of the axis and appears to be the elongation of the posterior longitudinal ligament.
- The alar ligament is made up of two strong rounded cords. Each cord begins at each side of the upper part of the dens and then passes obliquely upward and laterally to attach to the medial side of the condyles of the

occipital bone. Due to the origination of the ligament, it is lax in extension and taut in flexion. Its function is to limit flexion of the skull upon C1 vertebra and axial rotation of the head.

- The apical ligament is situated between the alar ligaments. It extends from the tip of the odontoid process to the anterior margin of foramen magnum.

The anterior atlanto-axial ligament, the posterior atlanto-axial ligament and the transverse ligament are the three principal ligaments in the C1/2 joint (Figure 6).

- The anterior atlanto-axial ligament extends from the lower border of the anterior arch of the atlas to the front of the axis body. It is thickened in the median plane and then tapped distally to form a round cord connecting to the anterior arch tubercle of the atlas.
- The posterior atlanto-axial ligament extends from the lower border of the posterior arch of the atlas to the upper edges of the lamina of the axis.
- The transverse ligament is a strong thick band. It links up the medial tubercles of the lateral masses of C1, encircling the dens. A thin layer of articular cartilage covers the median part of the anterior surface of the ligament. When the ligament crosses the dens, it divides into two small longitudinal bands. One extends upwards while the other goes downwards. A cross appearance is formed. Therefore, this is also known as the cruciform ligament of the atlas.

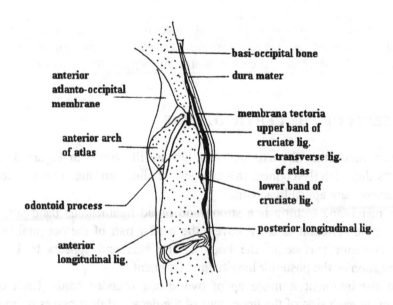

Figure 6. Ligaments of the atlanto-axial and atlanto-occipital joints.

There are also some important ligaments, which are general to the whole spine, including the anterior longitudinal ligament, the posterior longitudinal ligaments, the ligamentum flava, the interspinous ligaments, the intertranverse ligament and the ligamentum nuchae.

- The anterior longitudinal ligament is a strong ligamentus band. It extends from the occipital bone to the sacrum and covers the anterior surfaces of all vertebral bodies. The ligament is thick in the vertebral bodies region but relatively thin in the intervertebral disc region.
- Similarly, the posterior longitudinal ligament extends from the axis to the sacrum and covers the posterior surfaces of the vertebral bodies inside the vertebral canal. As compared with the anterior longitudinal ligament, the posterior longitudinal ligament is relatively thick in the disc region but thin in the vertebral body region.
- The ligamentum flava is located between the laminae of adjacent vertebrae (Figures 4 and 7). It extends from the lower anterior surface of lamina to the upper margin of posterior surface of lamina in the next segment. As this ligament is rich in yellow elastic fibres, it is known as the yellow ligament. It can both protect the spinal cord and assist in the control of spinal motion. In flexion, ligamentum flava will be stretched. Flexion of the spine will not be limited until the ligament becomes taut. In extension, the ligament will recoil in order to minimise the space it takes up inside the vertebral canal.
- The interspinous ligament is located between adjacent spinous processes and joins the ligamentum flava anteriorly and the supraspinous ligament posteriorly. However, this ligament is poorly developed in the cervical region. The supraspinous ligament extends from C7 to the sacrum and connects the apices of the spinous processes. This ligament can be roughly divided into three portions. The superficial fibres extend over three or four vertebrae. The intermediate fibres extend over two to three vertebrae while the deepest fibres connect the spines of neighbouring vertebrae.
- Intertransverse ligaments lie between the transverse processes of adjacent vertebrae. They help to limit lateral flexion and axial rotation of the spine.
- Ligamentum nuchae is fibro-elastic membrane. It begins from the external occipital protuberance and extends along the crest of the spinous processes of the cervical spine. It aids the attachment for neck muscles and strengthens the connection between the whole cervical vertebral column and the cranium.

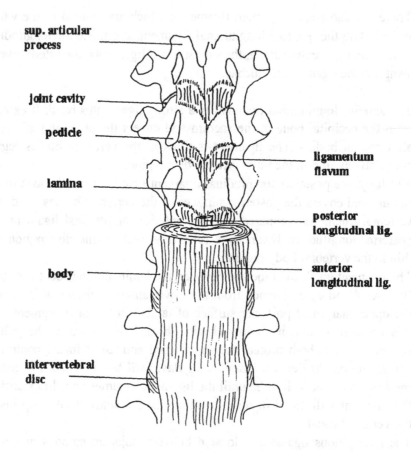

sup. articular process

joint cavity

pedicle

lamina

ligamentum flavum

posterior longitudinal lig.

anterior longitudinal lig.

body

intervertebral disc

Figure 7 Anterior view of the anterior longitudinal ligament and the ligamentum flava.

MOBILITY OF THE CERVICAL SPINE

The superior articular facets of the cervical vertebrae are posteriorly, superiorly and medially orientated. Flexion and extension of the cervical spine are generally unrestricted. However, the mobility of the cervical spine does vary within C1 to C7, due to regional variation of the anatomical structures of the cervical spine. The rotatory movement of the head is mainly provided by the pivot joint of C1/2 with an axis coinciding with the vertical axis of the dens. The extent of rotation is limited by the alar ligament. The types of movement permitted by the atlanto-occipital joints are flexion/extension (nodding) and a small degree of lateral flexion. Extension of the atlanto-occipital joint is limited due to a close pack configuration between the superior atlanto facet and the condylar fossa of the occipital bone. Similarly, extension of the lower cervical spine is limited by the interlocking configuration between facet joints.

Most of the flexion/extension motion occurs in the mid-cervical region. Flexion is facilitated by the cervical lordotic alignment, changing from convexity to concavity. However, flexion is restricted by both the spinal ligaments and the apposition of the projecting lower lips of the vertebral bodies (Figure 8). Lateral flexion and axial rotation are coupled motion. Lateral flexion will take place with rotation due to the orientation of the facets joints. Rotation is particularly free in the cervical region. A majority of axial rotation occurs at the atlanto-axial joint while the rest of the rotation takes place in the lower cervical region.

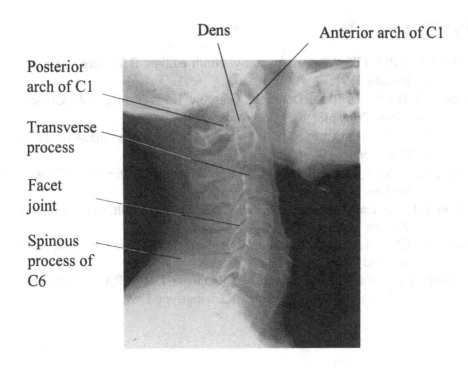

Figure 8. Lateral radiograph of the neck showing the cervical region of the vertebral column.

PRIME MOVERS OF THE CERVICAL SPINE

Muscles that produce flexion of the atlanto-occipital joints are anterior fibres of sternocleidomastoid, rectus capitis anterior, longus capitis. Muscles that produce extension are recti capitis posterior, semispinalis capitis, splenius capitis, longissimus capitis and upper trapezius. Muscles that produce lateral flexion are sternocleidomastoid, oblique capitis superior and inferior, rectus capitis lateralis, longissimus capitis, and splenius capitis. Muscles that produce ipsilateral rotation at the atlanto-axial joint are oblique capitis inferior, recti capitis posterior, longissimus capitis, and splenius capitis. Sternocleidomastoid muscle can produce contralateral rotation of the atlanto-axial joints. Flexion of the neck is produced by the bilateral action of longus colli, scalene muscles and sternocleidomastoid. Extension movement is produced by the bilateral action of splenius capitis, semispinalis capitis and cervicis. Lateral flexion is produced by unilateral action of splenius capitis and cervicis, longissimus capitis and cervicis, and iliocostalis cervicis. The rotation movement is produced by the unilateral action of splenius cervicis, multifidus, semispinalis capitis and cervicis, rotatores.

Suggested reading list:

Agur A.M.,GRANT'S Atlas of Anatomy. Ninth edition, Baltimore, Williams & Wilkins 1991.

Mathers L.H., Chase R.A., Dolph J., Glasgow E.F., Gosling J.A. Clinical Anatomy Principles. St. Louis, Mosby 1996.

McMinn R.M.H., Hutchings R.T. A Colour Atlas of Human Anatomy. Third edition, London, Wolfe Publishing 1993.

Moore K.L., Agur A.M.R.,Essential Clinical Anatomy, Baltimore, Williams & Wilkins 1996.

Moore K.L.,Clinically orientated Anatomy. Third edition, Baltimore, Williams & Wilkins 1992.

Snell R.S. Clinical Anatomy for Medical Students. Fifth edition, Boston, Little Brown and Company 1995.

Williams P.L., Warwick R., Dyson M., Bannister L.H. GRAY'S Anatomy. 37th edition, Edinburgh, Churchill Livingstone 1989.

CHAPTER 2

ESSENCES OF NEUROVASCULAR SYSTEMS OF THE CERVICAL SPINE

Margaret Kit Yi Mak

INTRODUCTION

This chapter discusses the internal morphology of the spinal cord and its relationship to the cervical vertebral column, as well as the nervous and vascular supplies of the cervical vertebral column. The discussion is based on information from Bogduk (1985), Cailler (1991), Gray and William (1989), Waxman and DeGroot (1995) and Westmorelard (1995). The vertebral canal of the cervical spine contains an important structure called the spinal cord. The cord is an extension of the brain projecting from the base of the medulla oblongata and occupies most of the vertebral canal. The spinal cord can be divided into five regions, including the cervical, thoracic, lumbar, sacral and coccygeal. It can be further subdivided into eight cervical segments, twelve thoracic segments, five lumbar segments, five sacral segments and a few coccgeal segments.

INTERNAL MORPHOLOGY OF THE SPINAL CORD

In a typical cross sectional specimen of the spinal cord, a deep anterior median fissure and a shallow posterior median fissure can easily be seen. These fissures divide the cord into left and right symmetrical halves that are joined at the central mid-portion (Figure 1). The cord contains grey matter and white matter. The H-shaped grey matter is located in the central zone of the cord and surrounded by white matter. The H shape is formed by the ventral grey column/horn, the dorsal grey column/horn and the lateral grey column which are bilaterally joined with a transverse grey commissure. The commissure is transvered by a central canal containing cerebrospinal fluid. Both the form and quality of the grey matter vary at different levels of the spinal cord. The

17

greatest ratio of the grey matter to white matter is in the lumbar and cervical regions. Therefore the spinal cord in these regions are termed as the lumbar and cervical enlargements.

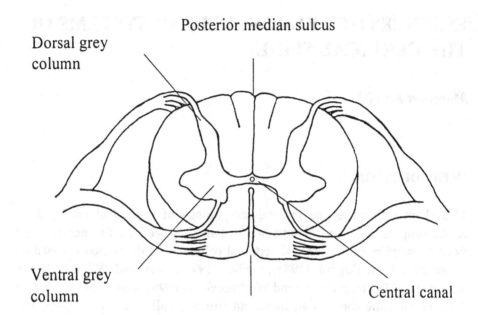

Figure 1. Morphology of the spinal cord in cross section
(adopted from Waxman and Degroot 1995:47).

Each segment of the spinal cord is connected to four nerve roots, including a ventral root and a dorsal root on the left half and a similar pair on the right half. The dorsal root enters the spinal cord via the dorsal grey column while the ventral root emerges from the ventral grey column. In the dorsal root of a typical spinal nerve, close to the junction of the ventral root, lies a dorsal root ganglion which is a swelling structure that contains nerve cells bodies. Afferent information of cutaneous and deep structures of the body are collected by the cell bodies in the ganglion. After synapsing with the neurons in the dorsal grey column, neurological information is then transmitted to the central nervous system through the ascending tracts in the white matter of the spinal cord. Efferent information from the central nervous system is conveyed via the descending tracts within the white matter and synapses with the motor neurons in the ventral grey matter. The motor neuron axons in the ventral root will then relay the neurological information to the appropriate muscle fibres. The distribution of the ascending and descending spinal tracts of the cervical spinal cord is indicated in Figure 2. Ipsilaterally, the dorsal and ventral roots in each level combine to form a spinal nerve, which is a nerve with mixed sensory and motor neurons. There are 31 pairs of spinal nerves in a healthy adult, including eight cervical, twelve thoracic, five lumbar, five sacral and one coccygeal spinal nerves.

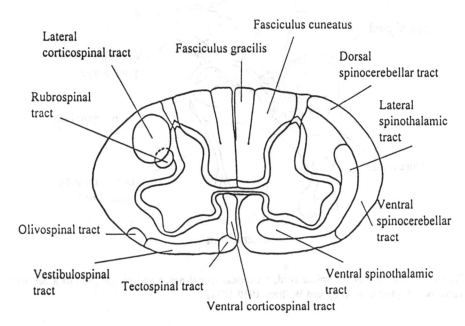

Figure 2. Major ascending and descending tracts in the spinal cord
(adopted from Gray and William 1989:817).

INNERVATION OF THE CERVICAL SPINE

The position of the spinal cord inside the vertebral canal of the cervical spine is illustrated in Figure 3. The dorsal side of the spinal cord faces the spinous process and the ventral side faces the vertebral body and the intervertebral disc. The dorsal and ventral spinal nerve roots remain inside the vertebral canal and do not extend beyond the intervertebral foramen. The dorsal root lies close to the articular process of the zygapophyseal joint and the ventral root is in close contact with the uncovertebral joint of the vertebral body. Having passed obliquely through the intervertebral foramen, the dorsal and ventral nerve roots of each segmental level unite to form a cervical spinal nerve. Viewing through the intervertebral foramen, we can easily see that the cervical spinal nerve and the nerve roots are bounded superiorly and inferiorly by the pedicle of the upper and lower vertebrae.

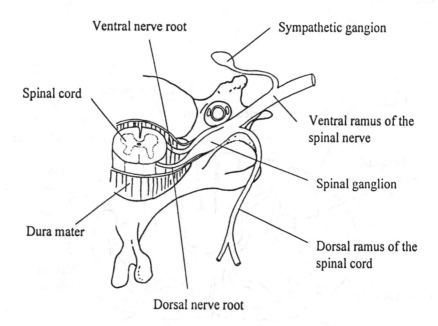

Figure 3. Structure of the spinal cord, a cervical spinal nerve and its ganglion to a cervical vertebra (adopted from Gray and William 1989:1031).

When each cervical spinal nerve emerges from the vertebral column, it passes through the intervertebral foremen at a level above the corresponding vertebral body. For example, the first cervical spinal nerve exits from the vertebral canal between the occipital bone and the atlas. It is therefore called the sub-occipital nerve. Upon departure from the intervertebral foramen, each cervical spinal nerve divides into two rami, the dorsal and ventral rami. With the exception of the first cervical spinal nerve, the dorsal ramus of the cervical spinal nerve further divides into medial and lateral branches to innervate the muscles and cutaneous areas of the posterior side of the neck. The medial branches of the cervical dorsal rami innervate the posterior deep neck muscles, including the rectus capitis posterior major and minor, the superior and inferior oblique, semispinal cervicis and capitis, multifidus, as well as interspinales. The lateral branches of the cervical dorsal rami innervate the superficial neck muscles, including the splenius capitus and cervicis, the longissimus cervicis, the longissimus capitus and the iliocostalis cervicis. These nerves also innervate the zygapophyseal joints of the cervical spines. The cutaneous branches of the cervical dorsal rami supply the skin over the head and the neck as indicated in Figure 4.

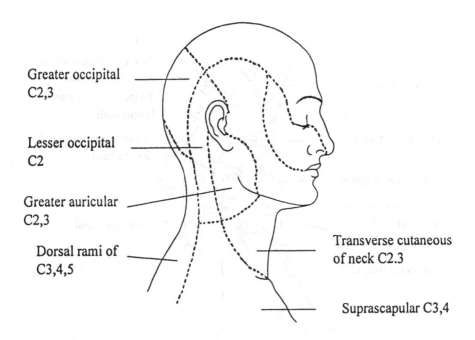

Greater occipital C2,3

Lesser occipital C2

Greater auricular C2,3

Dorsal rami of C3,4,5

Transverse cutaneous of neck C2.3

Suprascapular C3,4

Figure 4. The cutaneous nerve supply of the head and neck
(adopted from Gray and William 1989:1036).

With the exception of the first cervical spinal nerve, the ventral rami of the cervical spinal nerves emerge between the corresponding anterior and posterior intertransverse muscles. The ventral rami of C1 to C4 spinal nerves unite to form the cervical plexus. Conversely, the ventral rami of C5 to C8 join together with a great part of the T1 ventral ramus to form the brachial plexus. These two plexuses contain both motor and sensory nerves which supply most of the key structures in the neck and the upper limbs.

Cervical plexus

The cervical plexus divides into superficial branches to supply the cutaneous structures and deep branches to supply the pre-vertebral muscles of the neck, such as rectus lateralis, rectus capitus anterior, longus capitis, colli and sclenus, trapezius and sternocleidomastoid. The atlanto-occipital and lateral atlantoaxial joints are innervated by the ventral ramus of the first and second cervical spinal nerves respectively. The muscles supplied by the branches derived from the cervical plexus is shown in Figure 5.

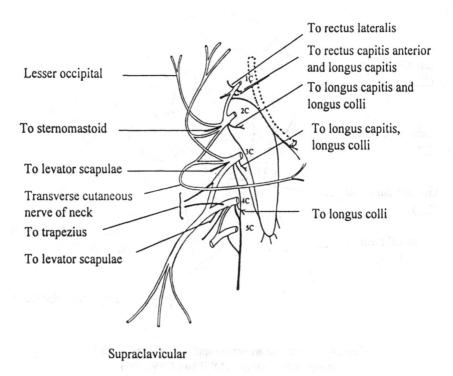

Figure 5. A plan of the cervical plexus showing the innervated muscles
(adopted from Gray and William 1989:1034).

Brachial plexus

The brachial plexus is divided into supraclavicular and infraclavicular branches. The supraclavicular branches further subdivide into the dorsal scapular nerve, the long thoracic nerve and the suprascapular nerve. Similarly, the infraclavicular branches further divide to form lateral, medial and posterior cords. The lateral and medial cord give rise to the lateral and medial pectoral nerves, median and ulnar nerves which mainly supply the flexor muscles of the upper limb. The posterior cord comprises of upper subscapular nerve, thoracodorsal nerve, lower subscapular nerve, axillary nerve and radial nerve. These nerves mainly supply the extensor muscles of the upper limbs. The plan of the brachial plexus is detailed in Figure 6.

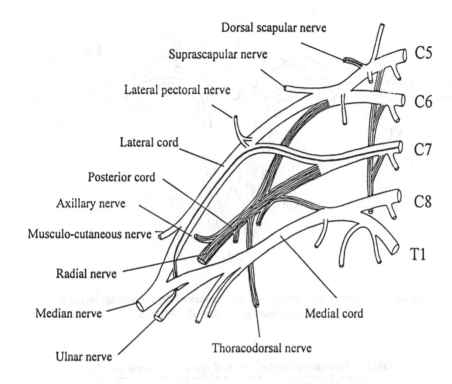

Figure 6. A plan of the brachial plexus illustrating the lateral, medial and posterior cord (adopted from Gray and William 1989:1038).

As a summary, the areas supplied by the eight cervical spinal nerves include the head, neck and upper limbs. The sensory fibres of each spinal nerve is distributed to its own dermatome, a well-defined segmental portion of the skin. The cutaneous innervation of cervical spinal nerves generally share a similar pattern with the segmental distribution of underlying muscle innervation (Figure 7). Myotome refers to the skeletal muscles innervated by a given spinal nerve. Assessment of the muscle and sensory functions can therefore be very useful to determine the segmental level with spinal disorders. Table 1 presents the muscles innervated by cervical spinal nerves.

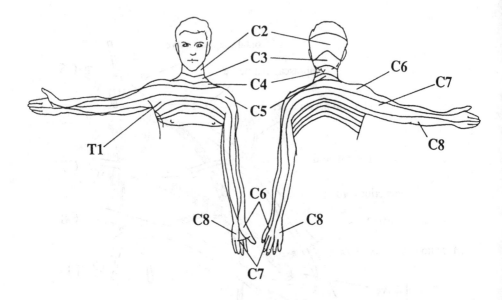

Figure 7. Segmental arrangement of dermatomes of the cervical spinal nerves
(adopted from Kandell *et al.*, 1991:716).

Table 1. Myotomes listed by cervical spinal nerves and muscles.

Spinal nerve root	Muscle
C3,4	diaphragm
C5	deltoid, biceps -
C6	brachioradialis
C7	triceps

SYMPATHETIC NERVOUS SYSTEM IN THE CERVICAL REGION

Two major components of the sympathetic nervous system are located in the
neck. They are the meningeal branches of the spinal nerve and the vertebral
nerve. The meningeal nerve, also known as the recurrent meningeal nerve or
the sinu-vertebral nerve, communicates with the thoracic sympathetic
ganglion. This nerve re- enters the vertebral canal through the intervertebral
foramen along the ventral spinal root and innervates the dura, the ligaments of
atlanto-axial region, the posterior longitudinal ligament, the posterior aspects
of the intervertebral disc, the periosteum and the walls of blood vessels. The
innervation of the anterior longitudinal ligament in the neck has not been
determined. It has been proposed to be similar to that of the pre-vertebral
muscles (Bogduk, 1988). The vertebral nerve runs along with the vertebral
artery in the foramen transversarium. This nerve supplies the lateral aspect of

the intervertebral disc (Windor *et al*, 1985). Irritation to this nerve may be caused by the mechanical pulsation of the vertebral artery anywhere along its course (Cailliet, 1991). Symptoms of vertebral artery irritation include headache, vertigo, tints, nasal disturbance, facial pain, facial flushing and pharyngeal parathesia.

MENINGEAL COVERING OF THE CERVICAL SPINAL CORD

The spinal cord is enclosed with three layers of membranes which are called the meninges. The inner two layers, the pia mater, are collectively known as leptomeninges. The thick outer layer is called the dura mater. A cross sectional view of the meninges and the spinal cord is illustrated in Figure 8. The pia mater adheres to the anterior side of the spinal cord and it dips into the anterior median fissure. It also adheres to the dorsal and ventral roots, as well as the dorsal root ganglia. Ligamentum denticulatum is a structure running from the pia mater to the dura. Its function is to keep the spinal cord in the middle of the dural theca. The ligamentum denticulatum has been shown to be useful to prevent the spinal cord from excessive elongation during flexion (Tani *et al.*, 1987). It can also relieve the tension of the spinal cord whenever there is excessive traction force in the cervical spine (Sunderland, 1974). Thickening of ligamentum denticulatum has been proposed to be associated with cervical spondylosis and this may imply cord degeneration (Bedford *et al.*, 1952).

Arachnoid mater lies between the dura and pia maters. The sub-arachnoid space, the space between the arachnoid mater and pia mater, contains cerebrospinal fluid. This fluid provides nutrition for the cord and can function as a shock absorber during sudden body movement. The pia mater communicates with the arachnoid mater via arachnoid trabeculae. Nicholas and Weller (1988) suggests that the arachnoid trabeculae may help to damp down the pressure waves transmitted in the cerebrospinal fluid during body movement. As the arachnoid mater ends laterally to the intervertebral foramen, therefore the cerebrospinal fluid will envelop the spinal nerve only up to the intervertebral foramen level.

The dura mater is a tough fibrous membrane in the outermost layer of the spinal cord. As compared with the neuroantary of the brain, it represents the inner layer of the cerebral dura mater. The periosteum lining the vertebral canal then represents the outer layer of that. This is separated from the spinal dura mater by an extradural space. The spinal dura mater is attached to the circumference of the foramen magnum and to the posterior surfaces of the bodies of C2 and C3. It is connected by fibrous slips to the posterior longitudinal ligament of the vertebra. The extradural or epidural space, which separates the dura from the bony vertebral column, contains loose fat, areolar tissue and a venous plexus. The subdural space contains a small amount of serous fluid. This allows the arachnoid to slide along the dura. The dura mater enables tubular elongation of the dorsal and ventral roots of the spinal nerves.

Since the arachnoid mater ends laterally at the intervertebral foramen, spinal nerves are wrapped solely with the dural sheath as they pass through the intervertebral foramen. A portion of the posterior longitudinal ligament that has turned into a fascial sheath runs laterally. This will become part of the dural sheath and then continues as the epineurium of the peripheral nerves. The epineurium sheath is firmly attached to both the transverse processes of the vertebra, the fascial prolongation of the posterior longitudinal ligament and scalene muscles. Since this sheath is firmly attached to the bony surface of the cervical spine, it helps to prevent the nerves from being avulsed from the spinal cord during a traction injury. A minimal angulation of the spinal nerves and the ligamentum denticulatum also protect the nerves from trauma or excessive stretching.

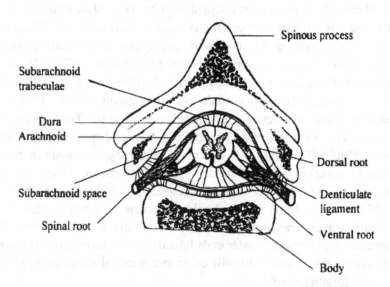

Figure 8. A transverse section of the spinal cord and its meninges
(adopted from Butler 1991:17).

Although spinal nerve roots cannot glide in and out of the foramen, some minute "up and down" movement of the nerve roots is allowed during neck movement (Cailliet, 1991). The posterior dural sheath is taut when the neck is in neutral position. The tension will increase when the neck is in flexion. The nerve roots will be pulled into a more horizontal position and occupy the uppermost position of the intervertebral foramen. As the neck is in extension, the dura relaxes. The nerve roots will slack into a more vertical position in relation to the spinal cord and lose contact with the inferior vertebral notch of the pedicle above. Since the cervical nerve root and its spinal nerve occupy only one-fourth and one-fifth of the area of the foramen on average, a small degree of movement in the spinal nerves will not cause any discomfort or abnormal symptoms. Only if the foramen is narrow (caused by either inflammation of the proximal joints, degeneration of the intervertebral disc or fibrosis of the body structures), will the functions of the spinal nerves be impaired.

BLOOD SUPPLY OF THE CERVICAL SPINAL CORD

The spinal cord is supplied by blood vessels that branch out from the vertebral artery and intercostal radicular arteries. Figure 9 illustrates the course of the vertebral artery going upward to the brain through the foramen transversarium.

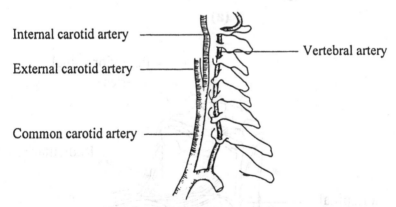

Internal carotid artery

External carotid artery

Vertebral artery

Common carotid artery

Figure 9. Course of the vertebral artery inside along the foramen transversarium (adopted from Kandell *et al.*:724).

The anterior spinal artery is formed by the union of the right and left bifurcation of the vertebral arteries. It descends along the ventral surface of the cervical spinal cord and supplies about 2/3 of the cross sectional area of the spinal cord. The ventral grey column and the base of the dorsal grey column, including the dorsal nucleus and adjacent white matter are covered. Posterior spinal arteries are another branch of the vertebral artery and their sizes are much smaller than that of the anterior spinal arteries. The posterior spinal arteries supply the dorsal white column and the rest of the dorsal grey column.

The nerve roots are supplied by the anterior and posterior radicular arteries. The arterial supply to the spinal cord is shown in Figure 10.

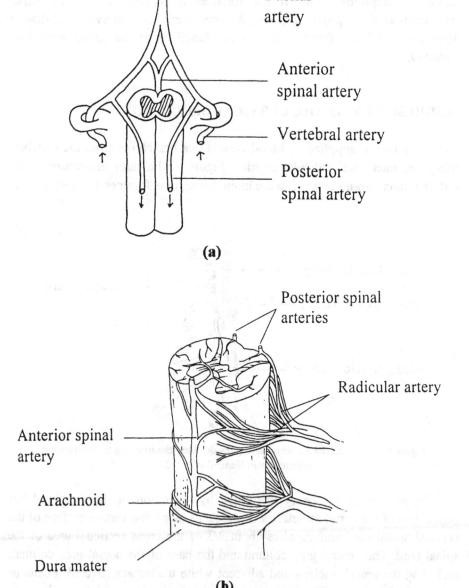

Figure 10. Diagram of the anterior and posterior spinal arteries at the spinal cord; (A) extrinsic arteries (adopted from Cailliet 1991:120), (B) intrinsic arteries (adopted from Westmoreland *et al.*, 1995:375).

Venous drainage is carried out by an irregular external venous plexus, which lies in the epidural space. This plexus communicates with the anterior and posterior spinal veins of the vertebral column. The venous return is ultimately drained into the vena cavae. The first and second cervical nerves are close to the vertebral artery, particularly at its point of angulation prior to entering the skull through the foramen magnum. These nerves are therefore vulnerable to irritation on injury. The common compression sites of the vertebral artery are at the sixth cervical spine, the atlanto-axial joint and the occipito-atlanto junction, particularly when the occipital condyle slides over the first cervical spine (Cailliet, 1991).

PHYSIOLOGY OF THE CERVICAL PAIN

Pain sensitive structures within the cervical spinal column are supplied by either the meningeal or the vertebral nerves. These structures include dura, interspinous ligaments, intervertebral discs, the atlanto-occipital and atlanto-axial joints and their associated ligaments, zygapophyseal joint and its articulation surfaces, nerve roots and neck muscles. A lesion in any of these somatic structures will cause localised pain. Stretching of the cervical nerve or its dural sheath may cause vascular circulation impairment and ischaemia pain (Bogduk, 1988; Cailliet, 1991). The ligaments, synovial lining and the capsular tissue of the zygapophyseal joints can also cause pain if they are inflamed or injured. Pain can originate from neck muscles. Sustained contraction of neck muscles can reduce their blood supply and accumulate waste products, for example lactic acid, and then produce muscular pain.

Nerve root irritation can also trigger off muscle spasm reflex and then cause pain. Pain caused by lesion in a somatic structure may be perceived to be produced by other structures in a distant location. This syndrome is termed as referred pain. For example, neck pain stemming from the zygapophyseal joints, ligaments, muscle or intervertebral discs may be perceived to be from the head, shoulder, upper limb and/or anterior or posterior upper trunk (Bogduk, 1988). This is because afferent information of the neck converges with other afferent inputs from the peripheral regions of the body in which they end upon the same neurons of the sensory pathways to the central nervous system (Kandel *et al.*, 1991).

When the foramen is narrow, due to the inflammation of the proximal joints, degeneration of the intervertebral disc or fibrosis of the body structures, the nerve function will be impaired. When the spinal nerves or nerve roots are irritated, compressed or inflamed, they can produce localised pain. Nerve root pain is thought to be caused by the generation of ectopic impulses in nociceptive afferents in the affected root (Howe *et al.*, 1977; Loeser, 1985). Severe compression of the cervical nerves and/or dorsal nerve roots will cause sensory and motor impairments, in the dermatome and myotome distribution of the affected nerves or nerve roots. For instance, compression of the sixth cervical nerve may cause parathesia and hyperasthesia of the lateral forearm, thumb and part of the index finger. Weakness of the biceps muscles and depression of biceps jerk may also occur. The parathesia and motor impairment are suggested to be caused by blockage of the conduction in axons and compression of the radicular vessels causing nerve root ischaemia (Bogduk, 1988).

Acute central spinal cord injury is a severe neurological syndrome that may occur after a whiplash injury (deceleration hyperflexion or hyperextension). The syndrome is suggested to be caused by cord contusion or partial transient insufficiency of the anterior spinal artery, a branch of the vertebral artery (Schneider and Schemm, 1961). The syndrome reveals more motor impairment in the upper limbs rather than in the lower limbs, according to the topographic arrangement of the lateral corticospinal tract. Sensory loss can occur especially in the somatosensation of the thoracic and lumbar region due to the involvement of lateral spinothalamic tract. When cord damage is associated with haemorrhage, the symptoms may result in cephalad or caudad and may even cause death. However, when the damage is oedema, the gradual return of the motor and sensory functions is possible.

References:

Bedford N. Degeneration of the spinal cord associated with cervical spondylosis. Lancet 1952;12:55-9.

Bogduk N. Innervation and pain patterns of the cervical spine. In: Grant R. ed, Physical Therapy of the Cervical and Thoracic Spine. First edition, USA, Churchill Livingstone 1988.

Butler D.S. Mobilisation of the Nervous System. New York, Churchill Livingstone 1991.

Cailliet R. Neck and Arm Pain. Third edition, Philadelphia, FA Davic Company 1991.

Gray H., William P.L. Gray's Anatomy. Third edition, New York, Churchill Livingstone 1989.

Howe J.F., Loeser J.D., Calvin W.H. Mechanosensitivity of dorsal root ganglia and chronically injured axons: A physiological basis for the radicular pain of the nerve root compression. Pain 1977;3:25.

Kandel E.R., Schwartz J.H., Jessell T.M. Principles of Neural Science. Third edition, Connecticut, Appleton & Lange 1991.

Loeser J.D. Pain due to nerve injury. Spine 1985;10:232.

Nicholas D.S., Weller R.O. The fine anatomy of the human spinal meninges. J Neurosurg 1988;69:276-82.

Schneider R.C., Schmen G.W. Vertebral artery insufficiency in acute and spinal trauma with special reference to the syndrome of acute central cervical spinal cord injury. J Neurosurg 1961;18:348-60.

Sunderland S. Meningeal-neural relations in the intervertebral foramen. J Neurosurg 1974;40:756-63.

Tani S., Yamada S., Knighton R.S. Extensibility of the lumbar and sacral cord: Pathophysiology of the tethered spinal cord in cats. J Neurosurg 1987;66:116-23.

Waxman S.G., DeGroot J. Correlative neuroanatomy. 22nd edition, Connecticut, Appleton & Lange 1995.

Westmoreland B.E., Benarroch E.E., Daube J.P., Reagan T.J., Sandok B.A. Medical Neurosciences: An Approach to Anatomy, Pathology and Physiology by System and Levels. Boston, Little Brown and Company 1995.

Windsor M., Inglis A., Bogduk N. The innervation of the cervical intervertebral discs. J Anat 1985;142:218.

CHAPTER 3

BIOMECHANICS OF THE CERVICAL SPINE

Sai Wing Lee

INTRODUCTION

The cervical spine has three basic physiological functions: bearing weight, protecting the neural elements and enabling the mobility of the head. It is, therefore, important to study the biomechanics of the cervical spine related to these physiological functions.

As the neck is the only bony structure supporting the head, the weight of the head will be entirely borne upon the cervical spine. Although the weight of the head is only 20 lbs. on average, the cross-sectional area of a typical cervical vertebra is around 6 cm². The compression stress in the cervical spine is therefore very high. In order to fulfil the weight bearing function, the material properties of the cervical spine should be very strong. The configuration of the cervical spine is another important factor, which help to counteract the mechanical stress as discussed in Chapter 1. As the brain stem and spinal cord are fragile, they are embedded inside the vertebral foreman, where the neural tissues are fully protected by the surrounding soft tissues and bony structures. The anatomical relationship between the nervous system and the cervical spine has been discussed in Chapter 2. As upright posture is necessary for our daily activities, particularly for normal vision, the unconstrained mobility of the head in relation to the trunk is crucial. In this chapter, the biomechanics of the cervical spine will be discussed and some fundamental concepts of spinal kinematics will be explained.

BIOMECHANICS FOR THERAPISTS

Biomechanics is a specific field of study of how forces interact with biological tissues (i.e. body parts). It can generally be divided into static and dynamic biomechanics. Although mathematics equations are probably the best media by which to discuss biomechanics, most of the contents in this chapter are not explained with equations. It is because this textbook is prepared for rehabilitation science students and therapists who may not be mathematical orientated. A number of technical terms and concepts in biomechanics will be discussed with simple examples in the following subsections. It is hoped that readers can appreciate how forces interact with our body, how the disease processes can affect the normal functions of the cervical spine and what are the implications of biomechanics to therapists.

BIOMECHANICAL TERMS AND CONCEPTS

Degree of freedom

Degree of freedom is an abstract term, which is commonly used to describe the number of potential ways of a rigid body can move around in space. For example, when a ball rolls in a straight tract (Figure 1), the degree of freedom is equal to one. This is because the ball can only roll forward and backward on the tract.

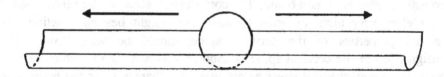

Figure 1. One degree of freedom of motion.

In Figure 2, the degree of freedom is two, because the ring can move up and down the pole and also rotate around the pole with an axis coinciding with the vertical axis of the pole. Picture a coin placed at Corner A of a table as in Figure 3. When the coin is moved from Corner A to Corner B, the degree of freedom is three. This is because the coin has been moved from left to right, from the lower end to the upper end of the table and also rotate in a clockwise direction on the table. Following this concept, for each functional motor unit of the cervical spine, except at the C1/2 level, the degree of freedom is six. This is because the superior vertebral segment of the unit can theoretically move upward and downward, forward and backward, side to side and rotate at the sagittal, coronal and vertical axes (Figure 4). However, it is important to remember that the substantial mobility of each functional motor unit is relatively small and the magnitude of movement may not be the same in different anatomical planes. This is due to the variation of the anatomical structures of the cervical spine at different levels and the mechanical constraints due to the surrounding soft tissues.

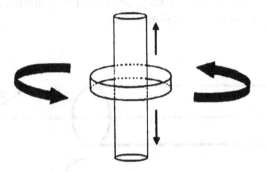

Figure 2. Two degrees of freedom of motion.

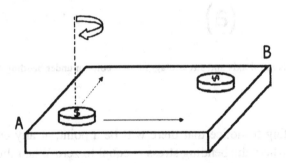

Figure 3. Three degrees of freedom of motion.

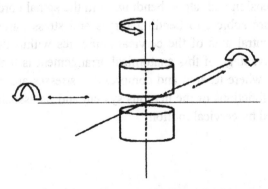

Figure 4. Six degrees of freedom of motion.

Cervical Spinal Disorders

Neutral axis

When a material is subject to bending forces, for example, when the two ends of a rod are bent towards each other as shown in Figure 5a, the materials in the upper layers of the rod will be in tension while the materials of the lower layer of the rod will be under compression. Stress developed across the rod will then gradually change from tension to compression. The pattern of stress can be illustrated using a stress diagram (Figure 5b).

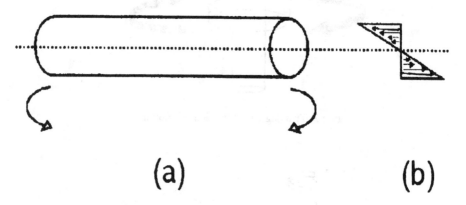

(a)   (b)

Figure 5. Neutral axis and stress diagram of a column under bending forces.

It is interesting to notice that there will be a point, at any cross sectional area of the rod, where the bending stress is equal to zero When these points are joined together, a neutral axis of the rod will be formed. The significance of the neutral axis is that the materials aligned in this axis are neither subject to tension nor compression.

In flexion/extension and lateral bending, both the spinal cord and the bony cervical column are subject to bending forces and stress patterns similar to Figure 5b. The neutral axis of the cervical spine lies within the spinal canal (Figure 6). The advantage of this anatomical arrangement is that the cord will be kept in a place where tension and compression stresses are minimal. Then, the physiological functions of the nervous system and its associated structures will not be affected by cervical motion.

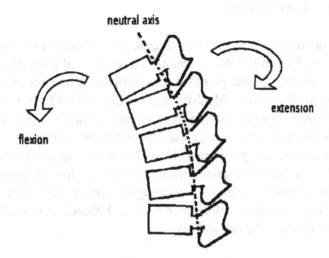

Figure 6. The neutral axis of the spine.

Instantaneous axis of rotation

When an object is rotated and displaced in air, for example a box has been moved from position A to position B in Figure 7, the instantaneous axis of rotation (IAR) is an imagined point where all the elements of the object have been rotated around this axis in specific moment. As the object changes its direction of motion in air, the position of IAR will then change from time to time. Assessment of IAR will therefore be useful to investigate the biomechanics of a joint, as in the designing of an artificial intervertebral joint. IAR of a functional motor unit of the cervical spine is located at the anterior portion of the intervertebral disc (White and Panjabi, 1978).

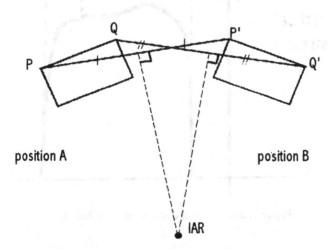

Figure 7. Estimation of the instantaneous axis of rotation of a moving object.

Intervertebral discal stresses

Stress inside an intervertebral disc can be generally divided into horizontal and vertical stresses. Due to the differences in the mechanical properties between annulus fibrosus and nucleus pulposus, the distribution of vertical stresses in an intervertebral disc varies. McNally and Adams (1992) have assessed the intervertebral discal stresses using a lumbar spine model. It is found that the vertical stress increases dramatically from the outermost surface of the annulus fibrosus to the inner margin of that. However, the stress remains relatively steady once it is within the region of nucleus pulposus where all points share a similar aquatic pressure (Figure 8). Although a similar study has not been performed using a cervical spinal model, it is believed that similar stress pattern will be found in the cervical discs.

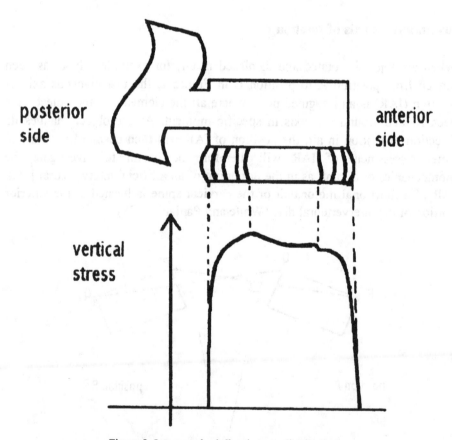

Figure 8. Intervertebral discal stress distribution.

Range of motion and pattern of motion

Range of motion is a general term to quantify the displacement of an object. It can be measured in length or in angle. Pattern of motion as defined by White and Panjabi (1978) is the configuration of a path that the geometric centre of the body follows as it moves through its range of motion, and determined by a combination of the geometric anatomy of the spinal structures and their physical properties.

For example, when a cart travels from A to B (Figure 9a), the range of motion is the distance between A and B while the pattern of motion is a linear motion. As compared with Figure 9a, when the cart travels from A to B on a trough surface, instead of level ground (Figure 9b), the pattern of motion of the cart will be a circular motion. Measurement of the linear distance between A and B can no longer completely reflect the motion of the cart. Angular displacement will therefore be assessed to denote its range of motion.

The implication of this example is that the validity of an assessment method of range of motion depends on its patterns of motion. Comparison of the range of motion should be only made when the patterns of motion in measurements are the same. If this assumption cannot be hold, the results of the comparison will be questionable.

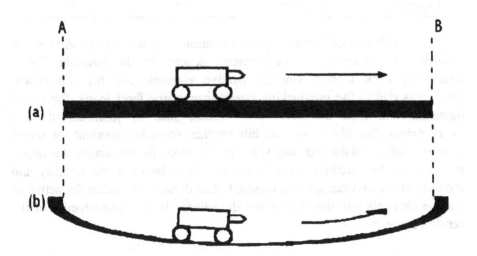

Figure 9. Comparison of the difference between range of motion and pattern of motion.

MOBILITY OF THE CERVICAL SPINE

As compared with the thoracic and lumbar spine, mobility of the cervical spine is generally the largest in all directions of motion (Table 1). The space available for performing extension in the cervical spine is larger than that in the lumbar spine. The average flexion/extension of the cervical and lumbar spine are 40° / 75° and 60° / 35° respectively. The significant difference in flexion/extension mobility of the cervical and lumbar spine is mainly due to the difference in the functional demands of these spinal regions. For example, a good extension ability of the neck can facilitate the visual function of the eyes when the head bends backward to look up at the sky; whereas bending forward is relatively important for the lumbar spine to facilitate sitting or picking up a pencil on the floor.

Lateral bending and axial rotation of the cervical spine contribute more than 50% of the whole spine in these motions. Therefore, a mobile cervical spine is significant not only for the head and neck, but also for the whole spine.

Table 1. Range of motion of the spine.

Regions	Flexion / Extension	Lateral bending	Axial rotation
Cervical	40°/ 75°	45°	50°
Thoracic	minimal	20°	35°
Lumbar	60°/ 35°	20°	5°

The mobility of the cervical spine is controlled by both active and passive elements of the spine. Active elements denote for the muscular forces controlling neck motion whereas passive elements are the mechanical constraints due to the interlocking mechanism of the facet joints, the spinal ligaments and their associated soft tissues, such as joint capsule and intervertebral disc fibres. As a mobile cervical spine is important for motor function while a stable cervical spine is important for protecting the neural elements in the vertebral canal, a good balance between the stability and mobility of the cervical spine is required. Any disorders in either the active or passive elements will therefore offset the balance in the biomechanics of the cervical spine.

MOTION DISORDER AND ITS ASSOCIATION WITH SYMPTOMS

Either due to pathological diseases or trauma, when the anatomical structures of the cervical spine change to a certain degree, it may affect the mobility of the cervical spine. The physiological functions of the cervical spine will then be affected, which may produce symptoms due to disturbance of either the mechanical or biological systems. For example, if the interspinal ligaments of the cervical spine have been torn in a car accident, the passive elements of the cervical spine will be weakened. Due to a decrease in the mechanical constraints to the cervical spine, the balance between the stability and mobility of the cervical spine may then be upset. The mobility of the vertebral segments will increase and the mechanical protection of the neural tissues will decrease. When the neural tissues are irritated, their neurophysiological functions will be affected and may cause symptoms (Figure 10).

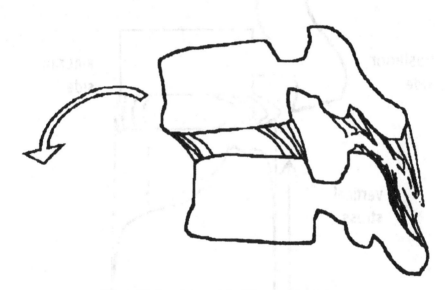

Figure 10. Torn intervertebral ligament due to trauma.

Similarly, when the anatomical structure of the cervical spine is weakened due to pathological disease, it may cause symptoms as well. For example, when an intervertebral disc degenerates, the water content of the disc decreases and the annulus fibrosus cracks. The discs may then bulge, which usually occurs at the posterior side of the spine. As one of the significant functions of the disc is to provide a movable joint between vertebral segments, a bulge disc will affect cervical spinal mobility. The distribution of stress (Figure 11) and the position of the neutral axis of the cervical spine may be shifted. Symptoms may then appear if the neurological system of the cervical spine cannot accommodate these changes.

In order to restore the physiological functions of the cervical spine, a number of therapeutic interventions have been devised to stabilise the cervical spine. For example, intervertebral fusion is a surgical method which can immobilise a pathological segment using either bone graft or internal fixators. Cervical orthoses are therapeutic devices which can be applied on the neck to increase the stiffness of the cervical spine externally. Specific exercise programmes may be also used to re-educate the deep neck muscles to provide active stabilisation effect for the cervical spine.

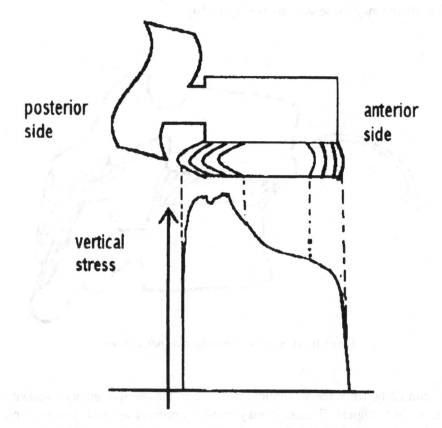

Figure 11. Increase of the posterior vertical stress in a degenerated intervertebral disc.

ASSESSMENT OF CERVICAL SPINAL MOTION

Spinal goniometry is one of the objective methods which is commonly used to assess patients with cervical spinal disorders in clinical practice. It has been also included as one of the assessment items in the evaluation of patients with physical disability. Assessment of cervical spinal motion is not only helpful in assisting therapists to make diagnoses with confidence, but will also be helpful for therapists in planning treatment and evaluating treatment outcome.

Cervical spinal motion is commonly assessed with a simple gravity dependent goniometer (Figure 12). The range of motion is then measured as the angular displacement of the head relative to the thorax. It can be alternatively measured as the change of distance between specific bony landmarks in the head and the thorax, such as the chin and the sternal notch in flexion.

The advantage of these methods is that they are simple and easy to apply in clinical settings. However, the reliability of these methods are only fair, as these assessment methods are relatively crude and cannot be used to assess the pattern of motion. If the pattern of motion of the patient has changed due to pathological disease, for example compressed fracture of C4, the value of assessing the range of motion will then be limited.

Using radiological methods, the assessment of the IAR of the cervical spine has been suggested to be helpful in identifying specific segments with motion disorders. A specific treatment plan can be then made. However, IAR is an error-sensitive parameter. The margins of error in IAR measurement are large and this affects its reliability. Moreover, as a non-invasion measurement method of IAR has not been developed yet, further studies in devising a practical assessment method are required.

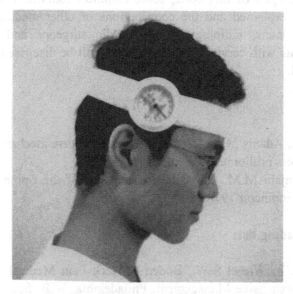

Figure 12. A Myrin goniometer.

With technological advancement, continuous assessment of the three-dimensional motion of the cervical spine has become popular since the 1980's. A number of commercial measurement devices have been developed and six degrees of freedoms of motion of the head and neck can be measured. Although the assessment results are relatively complicated, investigation of the changes in patterns of motion is possible. As a massive amount of data can be generated within a very short period of time using these modern devices, there should be careful interpretation of the data obtained so that the results can become meaningful to clinical practice.

SUMMARY

In this chapter, some biomechanical terms and concepts have been introduced. The clinical significance of studying the biomechanics of the cervical spine has been explained. Due to the physiological demands, the needs of a mobile but stable neck have been discussed. The association between spinal motion disorders and symptoms has been illustrated with some common clinical examples. The clinical applications of biomechanics have also been highlighted. It is hoped that this information will be useful to assist therapists in making physical diagnosis, selecting appropriate treatment and evaluating treatment outcome for patients with cervical spinal disorders.

In the next part of this book, some common conditions of the cervical spine will be explained and the contributions of other medical professions, such as physicians, radiologists, orthopaedic surgeons and orthotists, in treating patients with cervical spinal disorders will be discussed from Chapter 4 to Chapter 8.

References:

McNally D.S., Adams M.A. Internal intervertebral disc mechanics as revealed by stress proliometry. Spine 1992;17:66-73.

White A., Panjabi M.M. Clinical Biomechanics of the Spine. Philadelphia, J.B. Lippincott 1978.

Suggested reading list:

Borenstein D.G., Wiesel S.W., Boden S. Neck Pain Medical Diagnosis and Comprehensive Management. Philadelphia, W.B. Saunders Company 1996.

Goel V.K., Weinstein J.N. Biomechanics of the Spine: Clinical and Surgical

Perspective. CRC Press 1990.

Porterfield J.A., DeRosa C. Mechnical Neck Pain. Perspective in Functional Anatomy. Philadelphia, W.B. Saunders Company 1995.

White A., Panjabi M.M. Clinical Biomechanics of the Spine. Second edition, Philadelphia, J.B. Lippincott 1990.

PART II

Cervical Spinal Disorders
in Clinical Practice

CHAPTER 4

COMMON CONDITIONS OF THE CERVICAL SPINE

Sai Wing Lee

INTRODUCTION

Cervical spinal disorders are commonly seen in clinical practice. The significance of studying cervical spinal disorders is that this can assist clinicians to make diagnoses with confidence; effective treatment can then be planned and appropriate modifications in treatment can be made whenever necessary. Therapists can also appreciate the role of other medical professions in the treatment of patients with cervical spinal disorders. This will be helpful in strengthening the co-operation between therapists and medical professionals in the other related disciplines.

The conditions of the cervical spine can be generally classified into different categories according to their causes. For example, the conditions of the cervical spine may be caused by direct trauma, sports or related to one's occupation. The discussion of these specific areas will be further elaborated in Part III of this book. Cervical spinal disorders due to inflammatory diseases, infection, tumour, degeneration and congenital anomalies are discussed in this chapter.

INFLAMMATORY DISEASE OF THE CERVICAL SPINE

Rheumatoid arthritis

Rheumatoid arthritis (RA) is a polyarthritic disease and the cervical spine is the second most common area where it occurs (Bland, 1974). The exact cause of this disease remains unknown. Immunity disorders and infection are believed to be two possible causes. Patients with this disease are usually young to middle age. The incident rate of the disease is higher in females than in males.

The onset of the disease is insidious. Pain and swelling of peripheral joints are the common clinical signs and symptoms in patients with RA. These symptoms will worsen with activities and ease with rest. Due to the inflammatory process, synovial membrane of joints, including facet joints and intervertebral joints of the cervical spine, will thicken. Articular cartilage will soften and break down. Subchondrial bone erosion and joint deformity will occur.

It is important to remember that the inflammatory reaction of RA is not just confined to synovial joints, the synovial lining of tendon sheath will also inflamed as the disease progresses. The tendon may then weaken and rupture as it is subject to a sudden jerk of motion. One of the classic examples is the subluxation of the atlanto-axial joint due to a weakening of the transverse ligament. As the brain stem is located behind the odontoid process, it will then be subject to compression and produce symptoms when subluxation of the atlanto-axial joint occurs (Figure 1).

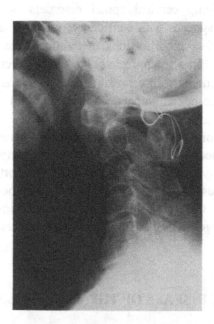

Figure 1. Wiring fixation of C1/2 subluxation in a patient with rheumatoid arthritis.

On clinical examination, the rheumatoid factor will be detected in the blood test. This antigen is known to be associated with the inflammatory reaction of the joint. Anti-inflammatory drugs are therefore usually prescribed to patients. A collar may also be prescribed in order to protect patients from subluxation of the cervical joints and provide the neck with a resting position. Patients are frequently referred for physiotherapy. The aims are to control neck pain and improve both joint flexibility and functional ability.

Although a majority of patients can be effectively managed with conservative treatment, some patients may not respond well to that. Surgical intervention will then be indicated. For example, ostectomy is a common operative procedure to correct joint deformity. When an inflamed joint causes unbearable pain, arthodesis may be indicated. However, joint mobility will be limited after fusion. Therefore, surgeons are required to balance the advantages and disadvantages before adopting this surgical option. Joint replacement is an alternative to fusion, particularly when joint mobility is crucial for patient's functional activities. However, the durability of prosthesis and complications of joint replacement remain to be the main limitations of this procedure. Synovectomy may occasionally be performed and the results are satisfactory.

Ankylosing spondylitis

Ankylosing spondylitis (AS) is another medical condition, which can cause an inflammatory reaction in the joints. This is particularly common in the axial skeleton. The pathogenesis of that is believed to be genetic-related. Most AS patients are young males aged between 15 to 30, rather than females. 95% of such patients will have HLA-B27 (histocompatibility complex) antigens.

The onset of the disease is insidious and patients will usually complain of pain or aches in the lower back and buttocks. Morning stiffness is a classic clinical sign of the diseases, but it can ease with gentle exercise. Articular cartilage, fibrous tissue of capsule and annulus fibrosus are commonly affected in the disease process.

On clinical examination, differential diagnosis can be confirmed with a blood test. Ankylosing signs can usually be found in sacral-iliac joints using plain radiographs. Following the ossification of spinal ligaments, intervertebral joints will gradually fuse up, leading to a "bamboo" shape of the spine (Figures 2 to 5). The resilience of the cervical vertebrae will then decrease and the spine will become brittle.

Subluxation of atlanto-axial joint and fracture of cervical vertebrae are therefore common when patients have a history of fall or direct trauma. The range of motion in the spine and peripheral joints will be progressively limited. Lung expansion will be restricted due to the rigidity of the rib cage. As a result, the cardiopulmonary functions of the patient will be affected.

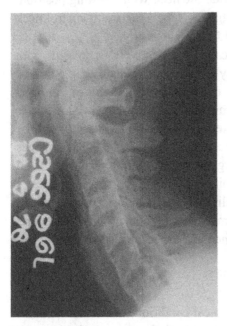

Figure 2. Lateral view of cervical spine with ankylosing signs.

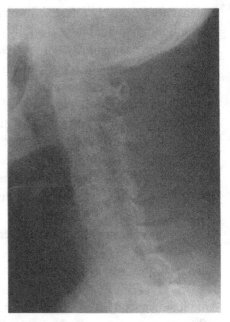

Figure 3. Oblique view of cervical spine, showing a decrease of intervertebral foramen.

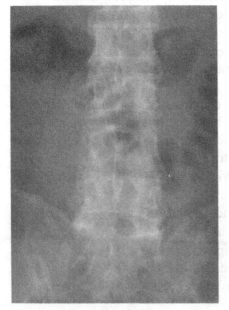

Figure 4. Ankylosing of lumbar spine with the involvement of sacral-iliac joints.

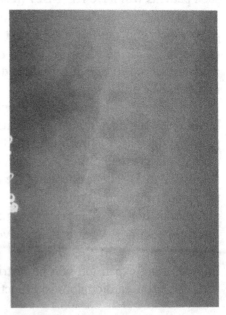

Figure 5. Ossification of anterior longitudinal ligament in patient with ankylosing spondylitis.

Therapists are commonly involved in the treatment of patients with AS. Different types of therapeutic means may be used to control joint pain when the patients suffer from acute exacerbation. Exercise therapy and occupational training are important to improve patients' joint range of motion and level of daily function activities. Active postural correction is necessary to improve the heart and lung functions, particularly in incorporating with aerobic exercises. Orthosis may be required to correct or prevent spinal deformity.

INFECTION DISEASES OF THE CERVICAL SPINE

Discitis

Discitis is the infection of the intervertebral disc. Staph aureus and pseudomonas are the common infecting organisms and their common entry pathway is via wound contamination. Reports of discitis are mainly related to extensive spinal surgery and discography (Figure 6). Patients with discitis will usually experience fever and complain of severe neck pain.

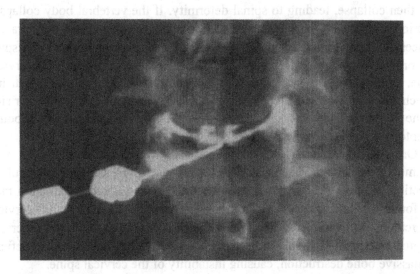

Figure 6. Injecting radio-opaque media into the disc, the integrity of the disc can then be assessed with plain radiographs.

Spinal motion is frequently limited. Decrease in intervertebral disc height may be found in the affected levels in the late stages of the disease process. Medical imaging techniques, such as bone scan, magnetic resonance imaging (MRI), may be required to locate the precise level of infection. Blood tests, such as white blood cell (WBC) count, erythrocyte sedimentary rate (ESR) and tissue biopsy examination, are usually helpful in confirming the diagnosis. Antibiotic therapy is the regular form of treatment for patients with discitis. However, if massive bone destruction occurs and affects the mechanical stability of the spine, surgical intervention may be required. In order to promote the healing of the spine, patients may be immobilised with a rigid type of orthosis. Details of different types of cervical orthosis will be further discussed in Chapter 8.

Tuberculous infection

Except in vertebral bodies, tuberculous infection in bone is uncommon. The infection pathway is mainly via the blood stream. As compared with the thoracic and lumbar spine, the incident rate of tuberculous infection in the cervical spine is relatively low. Patients are either children or young adults. Fever, neck pain and muscle spasm in the neck are the common clinical features of patients with tuberculous infection.

The anterior side of the vertebral body is a commonly affected area. As the disease process progresses, it may cause bone destruction. The vertebral body will then collapse, leading to spinal deformity. If the vertebral body collapses anteriorly, cervical kyphosis may be seen in patients' lateral plain radiographs. Abscess will be formed as pus discharges and accumulates between the spine and pre-vertebral fascia. If the abscess is in the anterior side of the cervical spine, it may cause compression of the oesophagus and pharynx, causing speech and swallowing difficulties. If the abscess develops at the posterior side of the vertebral body, the spinal cord may then be compressed and produce symptoms.

On clinical examination, an increase in WBC count and ESR will commonly be found. The Mantoux test is useful to confirm tuberculous infection. Radiological signs of bone destruction and abscess formation may be found in late stages of the disease process. Patients with cervical tuberculous infection can be treated successfully with antibiotic therapy. Surgical intervention is only indicated when patients have neurological deficits or massive bone destruction, causing instability of the cervical spine.

TUMOURS OF THE CERVICAL SPINE

Most cervical spinal tumours are due to metastasis. The tumour cells can primarily source from the spinal column, meninges, spinal cord, fibrous tissues of peripheral nerve or soft tissues in the cervical region (Figure 7). They are, however, very often malignant. As the tumour increases in size, the mass will then compress upon the surrounding tissues and cause symptoms. However, the nature of the symptoms will depend on the structure(s) being compressed. For example, neurological deficits may be caused if the spinal cord is compressed, and radiculopathic signs will be presented if the brachial plexus is compressed. In general, neck pain in patients with cervical tumours is usually localised. The pain intensity will increase at rest or evening. Tumours may cause bone destruction in the vertebral body, which can lead to compressed fracture or spinal deformity.

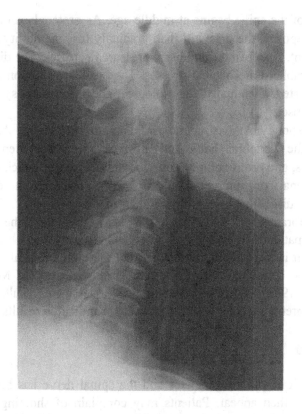

Figure 7. Sacroma is identified at the spinal process of C4.

On clinical examination, erosion of cervical vertebral bodies can be seen easily with plain radiographs. Radiotherapy and chemotherapy are the common forms of conservative treatment and the results are generally satisfactory. However, surgical treatment may be indicated as tumours cannot be completely controlled with conservative treatment and also if clear evidence of spinal instability is shown.

If the affected area is large, vertebrectomy may be indicated and the whole vertebral body will be replaced by fibular bone graft or a metal cage. Patients will then be immobilised with rigid type orthosis until the success of bone graft is confirmed. Physiotherapy may be required to maintain the physical condition of the patient during the immobilisation stage.

DEGENERATIVE DISEASES OF THE CERVICAL SPINE

Degeneration of the spine begins at middle age. As proteoglycan decreases in the nucleus pulposus, the disc will then gradually lose the ability to maintain its water content. As a result, intradiscal pressure decreases. The disc will then become vulnerable to mechanical stresses. The breakdown of annulus fibrosus will be accelerated. Eventually, the biological and mechanical systems of the spine will be upset.

Cervical spondylosis is a non-inflammatory disease. As the disc degenerates, the vertebral body and articular facets are then subject to abnormal stress, and proliferation of osteophytes may occur which may narrow the spinal canal or intervertebral foramen. Therefore, a decrease in intervertebral disc height, proliferation of osteophytes, decrease in intervertebral foramen or canal size are the classic findings in the radiological assessment of patient with cervical spine degenerative disorders.

However, it is important to remember that these radiological signs are not necessary to be correlated with symptoms (Friendenberg and Miller, 1963; Heller *et al.*, 1983). Therefore, radiological assessment results should be carefully interpreted together with the physical examination results of patients.

Radiculopathy

When the cervical spine degenerates and the spinal nerve has been irritated, symptoms may then appear. Patients may complain of shooting pain or an electric shock sensation distributed in the dermatome(s) supplied by the affected nerve(s). Patients may also complain of paraesthesia in hands and fingers. Neck motion may be restricted in all directions, particularly in extension, which will aggravate the symptoms. Weakness or muscle wasting in upper limb is relatively rare except in chronic cases. The reflexes of the upper limb usually remains normal.

Radiographs may be taken to rule out other conditions, such as fractures, tumours and infections. MRI will only be indicated if an operation is considered, although surgical intervention for a patient with radiculopathy is seldom required. Rest, analgesics, anti-inflammatory drugs and physiotherapy are the common forms of conservative treatment for these patients. A cervical collar may occasionally be required if patients are unable to establish a resting posture, particularly in an acute exacerbation stage.

Myelopathy

Cervical myelopathy is another type of non-inflammatory disease which is common in the elderly. The patho-mechanism is mainly due to physical compression of the spinal cord. The compression can either be caused by a degenerative disc, distension of the ligamentum flava, osteophytes encroachment, spinal deformity, tumours or instability of the cervical spine.

The clinical presentation of patients varies a lot because it depends on the nature of pathology, the rate of progression of the condition and the extent of spinal cord involvement. The onset of the disease is usually insidious. As long tract neurones embedded inside the spinal cord are affected, positive Hoffmann or Babinski signs will appear. Patients may also experience abnormal cutaneous sensation. The muscle power of the lower limbs will gradually decrease. As the disease process progresses, gait and balance will be affected. Clumsy hand and disorders in bladder and bowel control occur. MRI will be useful to identify the location and extent of compression.

Fortunately, the prognosis of cervical myelopathy is good. Physiotherapy and occupational therapy are useful to maintain patients' physical independence and even assist them to return to work. Only some minority of patients do not respond well to conservative treatment and require surgical intervention. Decompression with or without fusion may be performed to relieve the cord syndrome.

Bulging disc

As compared with the lumbar spine, the incident rate of bulging disc in the cervical spine is relatively low. The common affected levels are C5-C6 and C6-C7. The cause of bulging disc remains unknown. However, it is generally believed that the pathogenesis is associated with previous injury, which may lead to premature degeneration of the intervertebral disc.

As the posterior surface of the disc is reinforced by posterior longitudinal ligament and the ligament is pain sensitive, the patient will usually complain of sudden onset of sharp pain and muscle spasm in the neck as the disc bulges posteriorly. If the spinal nerve is involved, radiculopathy symptoms will appear. Similarly, if the spinal cord is compromised, the myelopathic syndrome will appear. Cutaneous sensation, muscle power and the reflexes of the upper limb may be slightly affected.

Radiographic assessment is usually normal. Evidence of a bulging disc can be seen with MRI. However, any interpretation of these results should be made with caution, as abnormal findings in MRI is common in asymptomatic population.

For treatment, anti-inflammatory drugs and analgesics are useful to control the symptoms, particularly in acute exacerbation phase. Patients can then be further treated with physiotherapy. Generally, the prognosis of bulging disc is good and surgical intervention is seldom required.

Instability of the cervical spine

Instability of the cervical spine can be caused by degeneration. As the ligaments, joint capsule and fibrous tissue of the intervertebral disc degenerate, they will gradually lose their strength. Excessive motion of vertebral joints will then occur. This can irritate the neural tissues of the cervical spine and produce symptoms (Figure 8). The clinical features of patients with cervical spinal instability are similar to those of cervical radiculopathy or myelopathy, depending upon the structures involved.

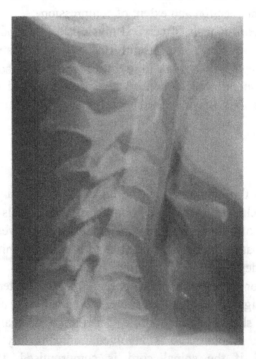

Figure 8. Instability signs are shown at the C4/5 level.

However, the diagnosis of spinal instability is relatively difficult. This is because patients seldom exhibit with a clear evidence of abnormal vertebral displacement even with MRI or computer tomography. The treatment for patients with degenerative spinal instability includes drug therapy, orthosis and physiotherapy. The aims are to provide support and symptomatic relief. Surgical treatment may be indicated if neurological deficits progress or significant functional disabilities are caused by the condition. Anterior cervical spinal fusion with autogenous bone graft is a common surgical technique to fix the neck. The long term outcome of this procedure is satisfactory.

COGENITAL ANOMALIES OF THE CERVICAL SPINE

Anomalies of the cervical spine can generally be divided into four types, including multiple congenital deformity, malformation in cranio-vertebral, atlanto-axial and lower cervical spine regions (Figure 9).

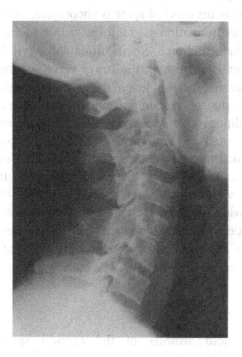

Figure 9. Cogential block vertebrae have been identified at C2/3 and C5/6 levels.

Down's syndrome is commonly associated with multiple congenital deformities. Although subluxation of the atlanto-axial joint may occur, spinal cord compression is rare. Cranio-vertebral anomaly is mainly due to malformation of the occiput. C1 and C2 vertebrae may shift upwards and protrude into the plane of the foramen magnum. The upward shift of the upper cervical spine does not necessarily cause symptoms, but patients with cranio-vertebral anomalies are frequently associated with congenital malformation of the central nervous system.

Anomalies in the atlanto-axial region can further be subdivided into atlas and axis anomalies. In the course of a clinical examination in the upper cervical region for other medical purpose, incomplete development of the anterior arch of the atlas may be occasionally detected. It is because this anomaly is usually asymptomatic. Anomalies of axis can be either related to the absence of the odontoid process or the incomplete fusion of the odontoid process with the C2 vertebral body. Surgical fusion may be required if neurological deficits appear or if evidence of spinal instability is found.

The Klippel-Feil syndrome is a benign anomaly in the lower cervical spine. The patient will usually have a short and stiff neck. Plain radiographs will reveal the absence of intervertebral joints.

Spondylolisthesis in the cervical spine is uncommon, as compared with the lumbar spine. This malformation is due to a failure of fusion between the vertebral body and the neural arch. Spinal bifida and cervical ribs are another types of development anomalies in the lower cervical spine. However, the incident rates of these are relatively low in the general population.

Having read this chapter, readers are supposed to have a general idea of some common conditions of the cervical spine. Full descriptions of these conditions can be found in any standard medical textbook. Readers are therefore recommended to read the references which are listed at the end of this chapter. Readers are also encouraged to understand their roles in the treatment of patients with cervical spinal disorders, instead of memorising the details. In the following chapters, the assessment procedures of patients with cervical spinal disorders will be explained. The diagnostic functions of medical imaging will also be discussed and the general principles of cervical surgery and the clinical application of orthosis will be introduced.

References:

Bland J.H. Rheumatoid arthritis of the cervical spine. J Rheumatol 1974;1:319.

Friendenberg Z.B., Miller W.T. Degenerative disc disease of the cervical spine. A comparative study of asymptomatic and symptomatic patients. J Bone Joint Surg 1963;4A:1171-8.

Heller C.A., Stanley P., Lewis-Jones B., Heller R.F. Value of x-ray examinations of the cervical spine. BMJ 1983;287:1276-8.

Suggested reading list:

Adams J.C., Hamblen D.L. Outline of Orthopaedics. 11th edition, Edinburgh, Churchill Livingstone 1990.

Bland J.H. Disorders of the cervical spine. Diagnosis and Medical Management. Second edition, Philadelphia, W.B. Saunders Company 1994.

Clark C.R., Bonfiglio M. Orthopaedics: Essentials of Diagnosis and Treatment. New York, Churchill Livingstone 1994.

Eurig J., McSweeney T. Disorders of the Cervical Spine. London, Butterworths 1980.

Macnab I., McCulloch J. Neck Ache and Shoulder Pain. Baltimore, Williams and Wilkins 1994.

CHAPTER 5

CLINICAL INVESTIGATIONS OF CERVICAL SPINAL DISORDERS

Raymond Ping Hong Chin

INTRODUCTION

Thorough appreciation of the medical history of the patient is of primary importance before any clinical investigation can proceed with direction and be meaningfully interpreted. Thus, it is common knowledge for clinicians that their thorough understanding of the patients' complaints, mechanism of injuries if any, past medical problems, and current medical status, are their first and foremost responsibility at the very beginning of the treatment process.

The goal of clinical practice is not only to tackle the individual patient's symptoms, but also to assist the patient to return to the community with an optimal quality of life. For this reason, information on the patient's quality of life, including his premorbid capacity to deal with the stress of active daily living and work, should also be taken into consideration. When treating a patient who is wheelchair bound for years, for instance, it would not be realistic to aim at independent walking.

Occupational history should also be considered because it indicates another important facet of the patient's premorbid life. To assist the patient to return to his/her own job is sometimes difficult, but it can be extremely rewarding. We need to know the nature of the patient's work and his working condition. This information can tell us whether it is possible to help the patient to return to his or her own work. And if he/she is considered to be able to return to his/her work, we need the above information to know how we can prepare the patient to take up the stress of his work again.

Since psychosocial problems may affect the clinical well being of patients with chronic neck and back problems, a good understanding of the patient's social history is also necessary. The common questions of clinicians on social history are:

Is the patient injured on duty? Is there any litigation involved related to the patient's clinical problems? Is the economical condition of the patient posing a great stress on the patient affecting his clinical well being? What is the condition of family support for the patient? Are we able to get any social support for the patient?

With good medical history, we can begin to plan our clinical investigations. We should not aim at turning every stone for information. In my opinion, the most efficient and effective way to begin clinical investigation of cervical spinal disorders is to do it systematically with defined objectives. The general objectives of clinical investigations are as follows:

1. defining and assessing symptomatology,
2. establishing a clinical diagnosis,
3. assessing the magnitude of the clinical problems,
4. obtaining further information to guide treatment.

1. Defining and assessing symptomatology

A majority of clinical complaints related to the neck is pain. Neck pain can be due to soft tissue injuries or other diseases that affect the integrity of the cervical spine stabilising mechanism. The pathology of the cervical spine causing neurological symptoms is usually identifiable by clinical imaging and careful physical examination.

However, pathologies of the cervical spine that cause pain may be quite illusive. Gore *et al* (1987) reported that neck pain can be associated with headaches, shoulder pain, arm pain, forearm pain and hand pain or numbness in 33%, 71%, 44%, 31% and 28% of patients respectively. Although the mechanisms of these referred symptoms are not well understood, the psychosocial factor in causing pain cannot be underestimated.

This is particularly important in patients with chronic pain who exhibit pain patterns that cannot be correlated to normal nerve distribution. Sometimes patients may complain of autonomic symptoms, like flushing, visual blurring, tinnitus, vertigo, facial numbness or pain. This can be related to the fact that there is autonomic contribution to the nervous plexus responsible for pain sensation in the cervical spine.

Nerve endings sensitive to noxious stimuli and responsible for pain sensation have been reported to be distributed in the capsule of facet joint, intervertebral discs and other soft tissues surrounding the spinal column (Bogduk, 1988; Cavanaugh *et al.*, 1995; Dwyer *et al.*, 1990; Mendel *et al.*, 1992; Rhalmi *et al.*, 1993). Provocative tests, such as injection of normal saline or contrast media into intervertebral discs, were performed by many researchers in order to identify the source of pain (Roth, 1976).

Anaesthetic blocks, using either steroids or analgesic, have been used to treat neck pain (Dwyer *et al.*, 1990). However, there has so far been insufficient evidence to support the claim that this approach can provide better longer term benefit to patients than the natural healing process. In 79% (Gore *et al.*, 1987) of patients with degenerative cervical spinal disorders, neck pain naturally eases with time.

Likewise for intervertebral body fusion, one of the treatment option to treat neck pain with degenerative intervertebral disc, the average success rate of surgery is merely 70%, which is actually slightly inferior to the natural healing rate of the disease.

In summary, both the diagnostic and treatment of pain over the cervical spine, are still challenging process for clinicians.

Neural compression syndromes

Neural compression syndromes (Heller, 1992) include radiculopathy and myelopathy. A comprehensive assessment should be performed in order to monitor the progress of patients. In Figure 1, a spinal cord injury admission form of the Queen Elizabeth Hospital is shown and the assessment items are detailed.

Radiculopathy

Radiculopathy is generally caused by nerve root compression around the intervertebral foramen, where spinal nerve root exits the spine. Intervertebral disc herniation is the most frequent cause in young patients. Conversely, osteophytes involvement are commonly found in middle age people and beyond with degenerative spines.

In general, pain produced by radiculopathy tends to be quite proximal in the upper limbs and may spread to other areas, such as the medial border of scapula. In contrast, paraesthesia is usually reported to be prominent in the distal part of the upper limb. The pattern of pain or numbness may follow the dermatome of the affected nerve root.

As overlapping in the dermatomes of different nerve roots is relatively common, interpretation of the clinical findings should be made with caution. It will be useful to correlate these findings with diagnostic imaging in order to identify the source of symptoms. This is particularly important when surgical intervention is indicated because an accurate localisation of the lesion is required for surgical planning.

HOSPITAL AUTHORITY	Hospital No.:
QUEEN ELIZABETH HOSPITAL	Name:
	I.D. No.: Sex: Age:
SPINAL CORD INJURY RECORD	Dept.: Team: Ward/Bed:

Date & Time of Injury:

			R	L	R	L	R	L	R	L	R	L
	Examiner:											
	Date/Time:											
* MOTOR			R	L	R	L	R	L	R	L	R	L
Shoulder	Deltoid	C5										
Elbow	Flex.	C5,C6										
	Ext.	C7										
Wrist	Ext.	C6										
	Flex.	C7										
Fingers	Flex.	C8,T1										
	Ext.	C7,C8										
	Abd. (intrinsics)	T1										
Trunk	Up abdom.	T5–T10										
	Low Abdom.	T10–T12										
Hip	Flex.	L1.2.3										
	Abd.	L4,5										
Knee	Ext.	L3,4										
	Flex. (med. Ham.)	L5,S1										
Ankle	Dorsiflex (Ant. Tib.)	L4,5										
	Plan, Flex. (Gastroc.)	S1										
Foot	Ev. (PL, PB)	S1										
Hallux	Ext. (EHL)	L5										
Toes	Flex. (FDL)	S1										
Rectal Tone												
** REFLEXES:	Biceps	C5										
	Brachioradialis	C6										
	Triceps	C7										
	Knee jerk	L2,3,4										
	Ankle jerk	S1										
	Bulbocavernosus	S2,3,4										
	Anal wink	S2,3,4										
	Cremasteric	T12										
	Plantar	UMN										

* MOTOR GRADING KEY:

5	100%	N	Normal:	Complete ROM against gravity with full resistance.
4	75%	G	Good:	Complete ROM against gravity with some resistance.
3	50%	F	Fair:	Complete ROM against gravity only.
2	10%	P	Poor:	Complete ROM with gravity eliminated.
1	0%	T	Trace:	Evidence of slight contractility with no joint motion.
0		O	Zero:	No evidence of contractility.
S – Spasm				If spasm, contracture, or injury limit ROM,
C – Contracture				place S, C, or I after the grade of a movement
I – Injury				incomplete for for this reason.

** REFLEX GRADING KEY:

0	No activity
1	Decreased activity
2	Normal activity
3	Hyperactive
4	Clonus

SPINAL CORD INJURY CHART

MR 0212 / QE

Figure 1. Spinal cord injury record chart used in the Queen Elizabeth Hospital of Hong Kong.

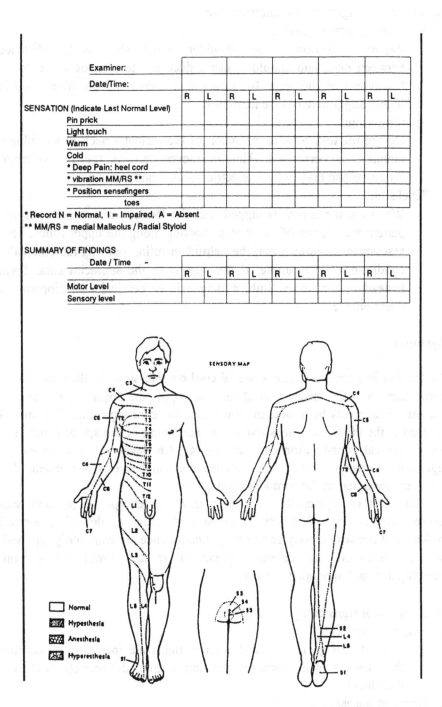

Examiner:										
Date/Time:										
	R	L	R	L	R	L	R	L	R	L
SENSATION (Indicate Last Normal Level)										
Pin prick										
Light touch										
Warm										
Cold										
* Deep Pain: heel cord										
* vibration MM/RS **										
* Position sensefingers										
toes										

* Record N = Normal, I = Impaired, A = Absent
** MM/RS = medial Malleolus / Radial Styloid

SUMMARY OF FINDINGS

Date / Time -										
	R	L	R	L	R	L	R	L	R	L
Motor Level										
Sensory level										

SENSORY MAP

Normal
Hypesthesia
Anesthesia
Hyperesthesia

Figure 1. (continued)

Useful physical signs for radiculopathy are:

a.   Shoulder abduction relief test

Passive abduction of the shoulder, which shortens the distance between neck and shoulder, can reduce the tension of nerve roots. Symptoms on the upper limb may then decrease. A positive result is highly suggestive of disc herniation.

b.   Spurling's sign

During the test, passive extension of the patient's neck in an oblique direction is performed. This manoever narrows the intervertebral foramens and may induce "electric shocks" and arm pain.

c.   Tinel sign

When the nerve root is tapped near the location of compression, the patient may report of numbness shooting along the upper limbs. This assessment technique may be helpful in ruling out non-radiculopathy conditions. For example, if the sign is in the supraclavicular fossa instead of the upper limb, a diagnosis of cervical radiculopathy is questionable.

Myelopathy

Myelopathy is a condition due to spinal cord compression. As there is a lot of motor neurons in the lower cervical spine to supply the upper limbs, the cord diameter is relatively large over the lower cervical cord segments. This area of the cord is therefore more sensitive to the narrowing of the spinal canal. The lower cervical spine, especially at the C5-C6 level, is also prone to degenerative changes, which may reduce the canal size to the extent that causes compression of the cord and myelopathy.

The onset of myelopathy is usually insidious except for patients with severe trauma. Gradual deterioration in gait, balance, dexterity, general weakness of the whole body and urinary incontinence are commonly reported. Pain is, however, not common (Crandall *et al.*, 1966) unless both radiculopathy and myelopathy occur.

Useful physical signs of myelopathy are:

a.   Finger escape sign

A positive sign is indicated when patients are incapable of keeping their fingers in an adducted position without deliberately stretching their hands.

b.   Grip and release test

This test is also known as the 10 seconds test. Patients are requested to grip and release their hands within 10 seconds. Myelopathy is suggested when there is poor motor control in the hands, so that the patient cannot grip and release their hands for more than 20 times in 10 seconds.

c. Inversion of brachioradialis reflex

Tapping on the brachioradialis muscle can induce wrist abduction reflex in a normal healthy person with intact C6 nerve root. However, this reflex will be suppressed when there is neural compression at the C6 level. Lower motor neurons below C6, such as C8 and T1, which initiate fingers movement will be blocked off from upper motor neuron control, so that finger movement will become hyperactive. As a result, finger flexion will be induced, instead of wrist abduction and, thus this is known as inverted radial reflex.

d. Hoffmann sign

This test can be performed by flipping the patient's thumb. If this causes flexion of the other fingers, it signifies that the patient may have corticospinal tract problems at or above C5 or C6 level. Bilateral Hoffmann sign may also be caused by anxiety or hyperexitability problems such as hyperthyroidism. On the other hand, unilateral Hoffmann sign when present, is considered to be highly diagnostic of myelopathy.

e. Lhermitte's sign

On passive flexion or extension of the spine, a positive result is indicated when pain and numbness shoots down the upper limb. This is due to the hypersensitivity of axons in controlling the nervous system when responding to mechanical stress. However, this sign is not specific to myelopathy and can be found in patients with radiculopathy or multiple sclerosis, etc.

2. Establishing a clinical diagnosis

Common etiologies leading to cervical spinal disorders include:

I   inflammatory diseases, e.g. rheumatoid arthritis and ankylosing spondylitis.

II   infection, especially in high-risk groups such as drug abusers or in patients with immune system disorder.

III   neoplasm.

IV   degenerative disorders.

V   trauma.

Other categories of diseases like metabolic diseases (e.g. acromegaly, gigantism, etc.) and congenital syndromes (e.g. Arnold-Chiari malformation, achondroplasia, Klippel-Fell anomaly etc.) are, however, rare in clinical practice. Inflammation is a normal immunity reaction and will appear as redness, swelling, heat and pain. These signs and symptoms are difficult to be observed in inflammatory diseases of the cervical spine because the spine is totally surrounded by layers of thick soft tissue, with only the tips of the spinous processes barely palpable.

One important point to notice is that pain resulting from inflammatory reaction is localised, as compared to pain induced by degenerative cervical disorders which is usually diffuse and vaguely defined. Fever is uncommon. Clinical laboratory tests can usually provide valuable findings. An increase of erythrocyte sedimentation rate (ESR) will suggest the presence of inflammation, though no specific location of the inflammatory process is suggested from a positive finding. An increase of white cell count can also suggest inflammation, especially using neutrocyte predominant white cell count.

Abnormal homeostasis in bone destruction and repair is another common pathology in cervical spine disorders due to infection and neoplasm. It can cause immense pain due to either the inflammatory process induced, impingement of fragments on nerves, or mechanical instability of the spine resulting from damage to normal bony architecture. The level of alkaline phosphatase can be assessed with biochemical tests. An increase of the phosphatase will then suggest an imbalance of the bone destruction and repair homeostasis. Again, no specific location of the pathology can be identified using the test. In spite of the lack of specificity, these tests are very sensitive and can prompt clinicians to perform further clinical investigations.

With the advancement of medical technologies, nuclear isotope scanning can spot an increase in blood flow or increase in inflammatory cells over the pathological lesion and helps to localise it. Diagnostic imaging such as computer tomography scans and magnetic resonance imaging can also provide multiple planar pictures of the human anatomy, as well as the pathological process.

Investigation of tissue samples, using specific techniques in microbiology and histopathology is also helpful in diagnosing of cervical disorders with infectious or neoplastic origin. Tissue sampling, however, is seldom performed in practice except during surgery, because percutaneous approach for the sample is difficult and dangerous in this part of the body.

3. Assessing the magnitude of the clinical problems

Cervical spinal disorders can cause physical impairment and affect one's functional capacity. It is, however, important to differentiate between impairment and disability because the degree of impairment is not necessarily correlated with one's disability level. Impairment, such as pain, motor weakness and numbness are the clinical manifestation of the inherent pathology. On the other hand, disability can be defined as the decrease or loss of capacity to deal with one's life and vocational requirement. The magnitude of disability is determined by a number of factors, including the demand of tasks, the presence of functional aids, patients' adjustment capability and the presence of co-existing impairment. The rehabilitation process plays an important role in modifying the effect of impairment over the patients' ultimate disability. The magnitude of the clinical problems can be assessed in terms of either the impairment involved or the disability resulting from the impairment. Using the spinal cord injury admission form in Figure 1, assessment of patients' neurological impairment can be performed. Neurological impairment will be assessed, pinpointing the three important functions of the neurological system, including sensory function, motor functions and reflex reaction.

Pain is a type of impairment that is difficult to be assessed objectively. A 10 points analogue pain scale is generally accepted to be a reliable method to assess pain. The dosage of analgesic consumed by the patient is another aspect to consider when assessing pain in clinical practice. Motor function impairment is commonly evaluated by the assessment of the patient's muscle strength and joint range. Work simulation is also commonly carried out to assess the patient's capacity to return to work.

In order to standardise the measurement and recording methods in assessing disability due to neurological impairment, a number of classification methods or scoring systems have been proposed to assess the magnitude of disability and evaluate the outcome of treatment. The Japanese Orthopaedic Association (JOA) scoring method is one of the common scales for the assessment of patients with cervical neurological disorders (Table 1). This scoring system provides a simple and quick measurement of the four important areas in patients with functional disability including:

1. motor dysfunction of the upper extremity,
2. motor dysfunction of the lower extremity,
3. sensory deficits of extremities and trunk and
4. sphincter dysfunction.

Due to cultural reasons, the JOA scoring system is frequently used in Asia because the skill of using chopsticks in feeding is used as one factor in the assessment of motor function. Nurick's Classification is another common measurement method designed to assess the physical disability of patients with cervical spondylotic myelopathy, with particular emphasis on ambulatory function (Table 2).

Table 1. The JOA scoring system proposed by the Japanese Orthopedic Association.

---

1. Motor dysfunction of the upper extremity
    0 = Unable to feed oneself
    1 = Unable to handle chopsticks, able to eat with a spoon
    2 = Chopsticks handled with much difficulty
    3 = Chopsticks handled with slight difficulty
    4 = None
2. Motor dysfunction of the lower extremity
    0 = Unable to walk
    1 = Able to walk on flat floor with walking   aid
    2 = Able to walk up and/or down stairs with handrail
    3= Lack of stability and smooth reciprocation
    4 = None
3. Sensory Deficit
    A. The upper extremity
        0 = Severe sensory loss or pain
        1 = Mild sensory loss
        2 = None
    B. The lower extremity, same as A
    C. The trunk, same as A
4. Sphincter dysfunction
    0 = Unable to void
    1= Marked difficulty in micturition (retention, strangury)
    2= Difficulty in micturition (pollakiuria, hesitation)
    3 = None

Table 2 Nurick's classification of disability in spondylotic myelopathy.

Grade	Description
I	Signs of cord involvement, normal gait
II	Mild gait impairment, ADL normal, able to be employed
III	Gait abnormality that prevents employment and normal ADL
IV	Able to ambulate only with assistance
V	Chair-bound or bedridden

4. Obtaining further information to guide treatment

Clinical treatment can be planned to either resolve the etiology of the condition or to relieve symptoms. Diagnostic imaging and neuro-physiological investigation are often useful to confirm a diagnosis. Authors including, Friedenberg and Miller (1963), Hitselberger and Witten (1968), Boden *et al.* (1990) have shown that abnormal findings in the medical images of the cervical spine are commonly found in asymptomatic population. These results suggest that the interpretation of these images should be made with caution and correlated with the clinical findings of patients.

As compared with pain, the results of neurological deficits assessment are relatively easy to correlate with medical imaging. Formulating treatment plans to deal with neurological problems is thus easier than dealing with pain alone. In general, surgeons are more aggressive in their decision making for patients with neurological impairment, especially for those with myelopathy. As neck pain heals naturally in a majority of the general population as discussed previously, surgical intervention may be indicated only when clear evidence is shown by a provocative test. Water-soluble contrast media can be injected into the intervertebral disc to provoke discogenic pain and to show discrepancy in the integrity of the disc using fluoroscopy investigation. The reliability of this approach is, however, controversial. Diagnostic imaging, e.g. x-ray, MRI, CT scan etc., besides assisting us in formulating a diagnosis, also give valuable guidance to surgeons in making clinical decisions in terms of surgery. In general, surgery serves three purposes in the cervical spine:

1. decompressing neurological tissues;
2. stabilising unstable spine segments;
3. obtaining tissue to establish a diagnosis.

The multi-planar images offered from the above state of the art technology tell us where neurological tissue is compressed, where instability is suspected, and which surgical approach is most appropriate for our surgical objectives.

AUTHOR'S COMMENTS:

Being a surgeon, I used to think that the single most important decision in the whole process of clinical investigation is to decide if surgical intervention is indicated or not. As years go by, I have learnt from my colleagues of other disciplines that surgery is not the only treatment option and certainly may not be the best option. This is especially true in treating patients with either cervical spine or lumbar spine disorders. I believe that making referrals to appropriate specialists is one of the most powerful tools in performing "clinical investigations". Whenever an MRI or a CT scan is required, we can make referrals to radiologists. Likewise, we can make referrals to physiotherapists, occupational therapists, orthotists, clinical psychologists, social workers and other related disciplines for their advice and assistance whenever and whatever professional healthcare services issues come up.

Making referrals is probably a mixture of art and science. This is because you need to understand the limitation of your own discipline and learn to appreciate and respect the contribution of the other disciplines. The ultimate aim of referring patients is to provide them with a complete and multidisciplinary medical care. Our patients will then be benefited beyond the capacity of a single discipline. Conversely, taking referrals should also be viewed as a process of understanding and respect. Active liaison and cooperation between disciplines should be initiated as required. As a clinician in the rehabilitation field, I think multidiscipline approach in treating patients with cervical spinal disorders is not an option, but a necessity.

References:

Boden S.D., McCowin P.R., Davis D.O., *et al*. Abnormal magnetic resonance scans of the cervical spine in asymptomatic subjects. J Bone Joint Surg 1990;72(A):1178-84.

Bogduk N. The cervical zygapophyeal joints as a source of neck pain. Spine 1988;13:2-8.

Cavanaugh J.M. *et al*. Innervation of the Rabbit lumbar intervertebral disc and posterior longitudinal ligament. Spine 1995;20:2080-5.

Crandall P.H., Batzdorf U. Cervical spondylotic myelopathy. J Neurosurg. 1966;25:57-66.

Dwyer A., Aprill C., Bogduk N. Cervical zygapophyseal joint pain patterns. A study in normal volunteers. Spine 1990;15:453-7.

Friedenberg Z.B., Miller W.T. Degenerative disc disease of the cervical spine. J Bone Joint Surg 1963;45:1171-8.

Gore D.R., Sepic S.B., Gardner G.M. Neck pain: A long-term follow up of 205 patients. Spine 1987;12:1-5.

Heller J.G. The syndromes of degenerative cervical disease. Orthop Clin North Am 1992;23:381-94.

Hitselberger W.E., Witten R.M. Abnormal myelograms in asymptomatic patients. J Neurosurg 1968;28:204-6.

Mendel T. *et al*. Neural elements in human cervical intervertebral discs. Spine 1992;17:132-5.

Rhalmi S. *et al*. Immunohistochemical study of nerves in lumbar spine ligaments. Spine 1993;18:264-7.

Roth D.A. Cervical analgesic discography: A new test for definitive diagnosis of the painful-disk syndrome. JAMA 1976;235:1713-4.

Suggested reading list:

LaRocca H. A taxonomy of chronic pain syndromes. 1991 Presidential Address, Cervical Spine Research Society Annual Meeting, December 5, 1991. Spine 1992 Supl: S344-55.

LaRocca H. Cervical spondylotic myelopathy: Natural history. Spine 1988;13:854-5.

Lee F., Turner J.W.A. Natural history and prognosis of cervical spondylosis. BMJ 1963;2:1607-10.

Melzack R., Wall P.W. Pain mechanism: A new theory. Science 1965;150:971.

Rothman R.H., Rashbaum R.F. Pathogenesis of signs and symptoms of cervical disc degeneration. AAOS Instructional Course Lectures 1978;27:203-15.

Symon L., Lavender P. The surgical treatment of cervical spondylotic myelopathy. Neurology 1967;17:117-27.

Torg J.S. *et al.* Cervical cord neurapraxia: classification, pathomechanics, morbidity, and management guidelines. J Neurosurg 1997.

Whitecloud T.S., Seago R.A. Cervical discogenic syndrome: Results of operative intervention in patients with positive discography. Spine 1987;12:313-6.

CHAPTER 6

DIAGNOSTIC IMAGING OF THE CERVICAL SPINE

James F. Griffith

INTRODUCTION

The past two decades have witnessed a remarkable progress in cervical spine imaging largely due to the advent of computed tomography (CT) and magnetic resonance imaging (MRI). These two modalities can demonstrate the bony elements of the cervical spine, the supporting soft tissues, the contents of the spinal canal, the cervical cord and the cervical nerve roots like never before. Prior to this, since the discovery of x-rays by Roentgen in 1895, imaging of the cervical spine was confined to radiographs. This in itself was a great leap forward, as before the discovery of x-rays, there was no means available by which to non-invasively look at the cervical spine. Hence, we have truly entered exciting times as far as cervical imaging is concerned. A good clinical history and physical examination is the key to correct diagnosis for most patients. And a correct diagnosis is the key to a correct treatment. The role of investigative imaging studies lies in confirming the clinical diagnosis and excluding other diseases which may produce similar clinical symptoms and signs. It is thus essential to interpret imaging studies only in the light of clinical findings. For example, if image studies show a possible tumour within the vertebrae but the clinical picture indicates an infection, then the possibility of acute osteomyelitis should be considered in lieu of a tumour (Figure 1).

RADIOGRAPHS

Radiographs are the workhorse of cervical imaging and will be the first line of investigation in patients with neck pain or injury. A radiograph of the cervical spine is taken by placing an unexposed radiograph ("x-ray film") within a cassette alongside the patient's neck (Figure 2). The x-ray tube, placed opposite, produces a parallel beam of x-rays. These x-rays will be absorbed to varying degrees as they pass through the patient's neck. Dense structures such as bone will absorb a lot of rays whereas less dense structures such as the soft tissues will absorb little. The amount and distribution of x-rays transmitted exposes an imprint of the patient's cervical spine on the radiograph. This radiograph is then developed in the x-ray darkroom producing a permanent image.

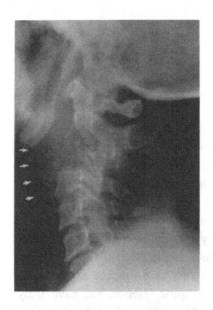

Figure 1. Lateral radiograph of cervical spine. This shows destruction of the body of C3 and the inferior aspect of C2. There is a large soft tissue mass anteriorly (arrows). These findings could be due to either infection or malignancy. There was no clinical evidence of infection. The final diagnosis was a metastatic deposit from lung carcinoma.

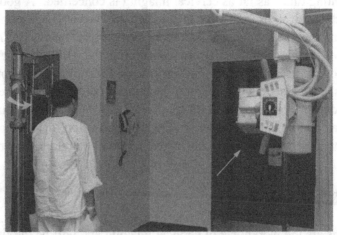

Figure 2a. Obtaining a lateral cervical spine radiograph. The patient is positioned close to the x-ray cassette (curved arrow) and away from the x-ray tube (straight arrow). Note how the patient is holding two large water containers to keep his shoulders depressed.

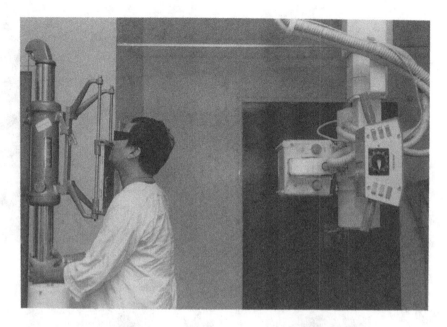

Figure 2b. Obtaining an antero-posterior cervical spine radiograph.

In order to view different anatomical areas of the cervical spine, radiographs are usually taken in more than one direction. A standard radiographic series of the cervical spine consists of a lateral projection (Figure 3a), an anteroposterior projection of C3 to T1 (Figure 3b) and, if pathology in the upper cervical spine is suspected, an anteroposterior projection of C1 and C/2 ("open mouth view") (Figure 3c). A less commonly used projection is the oblique projection (Figure 3d). This allows a good view of the neural foramina.

The lateral projection (Figure 3a) allows appreciation of the smooth curves formed by the anterior ("anterior vertebral line") and posterior ("posterior vertebral line") margins of the vertebral bodies and the junctions of the lamina and the spinous processes (the "spinolaminal line"). The area between the posterior vertebral line and the spinolaminal line houses the spinal canal.

The discs and other soft tissues cannot be seen directly but the height of the disc can be predicted from the distance between the vertebral bodies. Disc height should be the same at each level. Any reduction in disc height usually means established disc degeneration at that level (Figure 3a). As the degenerative disc bulges outside the margins of the adjacent vertebral bodies, it often leads to the formation of bony outgrowths at the margins of the vertebral bodies ("marginal osteophytosis") (Figures 4a and 4b).

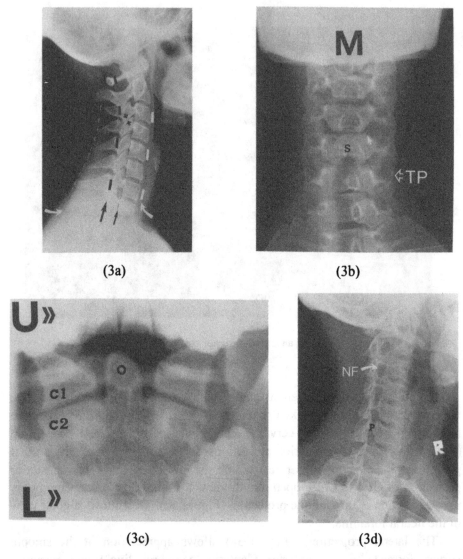

(3a)   (3b)

(3c)   (3d)

Figure 3a. Lateral radiograph of cervical spine. Note the smooth lines formed by the anterior and posterior edges of the vertebral bodies, the junction of the lamina and the spinous processes and the tips of the spinous processes. Note how all the vertebral from C1 to C7 can be seen. There is reduced disc height at C5/6 and, to a lesser extent, at C4/5 indicating degenerative disease. Small arrows indicate the facet joints between C3 and C4.

Figure 3b. Anteroposterior radiograph of normal cervical spine. Note how C1 and C2 cannot be seen as the mandible (M) overlies the upper cervical spine. The arrow points to an uncinate process. These are present at the supero-lateral corner of each cervical vertebrae from C3 to C7. TP = transverse process. S= spinous process.

Figure 3c. Anteroposterior radiograph of normal C1/2 ("open-mouth" view). Note the upper (U) and lower (L) teeth. O = odontoid peg, C1 = lateral mass of C1, C2 = lateral mass of C2.

Figure 3d. Oblique radiograph of normal cervical spine. These views are taken in order to look at the pedicles (P) or the neural foramina (NF). They are less frequently performed nowadays since the advent of CT and MR.

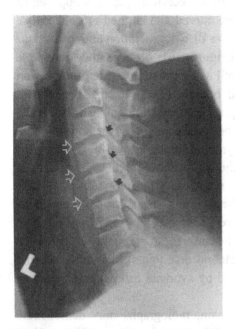 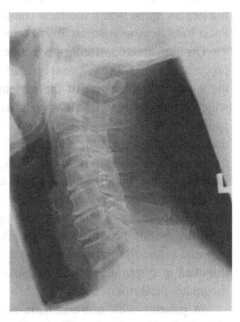

Figure 4a. Lateral cervical spine radiograph showing early disc degeneration with very mild reduction in disc height at C3/4, C4/5 and C5/6 (white arrows) in association with early posterior marginal osteophytosis at some levels (black arrows). Note also how the cervical spine in not as curved as usual (this is due to spasm of the paravertebral muscles)

Figure 4b. Lateral cervical spine radiograph showing severe disc degeneration at C4/5 and C5/6. Note severe reduction in disc height and mild posterior movement (subluxation) of one vertebra relative to the vertebra below (arrows). Posterior osteophytosis is not a feature of this case.

Although marginal osteophytosis can occur anywhere round the vertebral rim, osteophytes protruding posteriorly or posterolaterally are the most important since these osteophytes may impinge either upon the spinal cord within the spinal canal or on the cervical nerve roots as they emerge through the neural foramina. Therefore, pay particular attention to the posterior margins of the discs on the lateral projection. The other cause of reduced disc space height is infection within the disc ("discitis"). This can generally be distinguished from degenerative disc disease as infection will destroy the adjacent vertebral endplates whereas degenerative disease will not. The integrity of the supporting musculo-ligamentous structures can be predicted from the alignment of the vertebral bodies to each other (Figure 5a). On the lateral projection, also observe the facet joints. In the cervical spine, the facets are flat and at an angle of about 45 degrees to the vertebrae, thereby conferring a greater degree of flexion and extension to the cervical spine (as opposed to the lumbar spine where the facet joints are curved and aligned more steeply). Facet joint degeneration usually accompanies disc degeneration and visa versa.

On the anteroposterior projection (Figure 3b), observe the transverse processes of the C3 to C7 vertebrae, as well as the small uncinate processes on the superolateral aspects of the vertebral bodies. These uncinate processes, which are only found in the cervical region, confer additional stability to the spine, limiting sideways movement of one vertebral body on another. The uncinate processes are the site of small synovial joints (known by a variety of names, such as the uncovertebral joints, the neurocentral joints, or the joints of Luskha). These small synovial joints are noteworthy for two reasons. Firstly, if degenerative change develops in these joints, because of their close relationship to the neural foramina, any resultant osteophytosis may impinge upon the exiting nerve roots. Secondly, because these are synovial joints (as opposed to the fibrocartilaginous intervertebral disc joints), they may become inflamed in systemic diseases characterised by synovial inflammation such as rheumatoid arthritis.

In patients with non-traumatic neck pain, radiographs may demonstrate chronic disc degeneration (Figures 4a and 4b), metastatic disease (Figure 1) or infection. In acute cervical disc prolapse radiographs may be normal, particularly in young patients. This is because the main radiographic signs of degenerative disc disease namely (i) reduction in disc space height and (ii) marginal osteophytosis (i.e. bony outgrowths at the margins of the vertebral bodies) take time to form. It should be remembered that degenerative changes in the cervical spine will be seen on radiographs in most patients over forty years of age and the majority of these patients will be asymptomatic. So if a middle-aged or elderly patient complains of neck pain and the radiograph shows degeneration, this is to be expected. It cannot be concluded that the degeneration is the cause of the pain. If clinical signs are atypical, a further cause for pain should be sought.

The significance of abnormalities detected on imaging studies should always be correlated with the patient's symptoms. For example, in degenerative cervical spinal disease, modern imaging techniques will show abnormalities which are symptomatic in one patient while similar abnormalities are entirely asymptomatic in another patient. Hence the frequently heard battle cry of orthopaedic surgeons ~ "treat the patient's symptoms and not the x-rays!"

Disc degeneration most often causes pain as a result of compression of the exiting nerve root or the spinal cord. Less frequently degenerative discs can give rise to pain even without nerve root compression. This pain which is known as "discogenic" pain (i.e. arising in the disc) occurs as a result of radial tears occurring in the disc annulus as the disc degenerates. Usually many discs in a row will show signs of disease degeneration. It can be difficult to decide which disc is causing the pain. One way to solve this is to inject each disc in turn with contrast medium under fluoroscopic (i.e. x-ray) screening and see if this gives rise to the patient's pain. This investigation is known as "provocation discography". Whilst it is of some benefit in the lumbar region, it is of less benefit in the cervical spine as a lot of overlap exists between pain dermatomes in the cervical region. Moreover, provocation discography is painful and may lead to disc infection. Therefore it is not commonly performed.

Following trauma, radiographs help in the assessment of cervical spine alignment (Figure 5a), vertebral fracture (Figure 5b) and stability. Following severe cervical trauma, cervical spine movement is kept to a minimal and the neck is kept immobilised in a collar until radiographs are obtained. These help exclude spinal fracture, dislocation or subluxation (partial dislocation). If the cervical spine shows no evidence of injury on radiographs then the neck can be gently mobilised. If spinal instability is suspected, it can be assessed further by flexion and extension views.

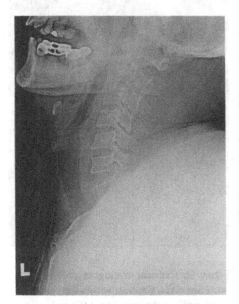 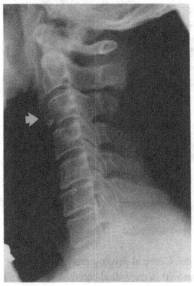

Figure 5a. Lateral cervical spine radiograph. This patient was brought to A&E department following a fall from a motorbike. There is severe widening of the C6/7 disc space. This could only have happened following severe hyperextension injury and indicates that the anterior longitudinal ligament is completely torn at this level.

Figure 5b. Lateral cervical spine radiograph following trauma. There is a small chip fracture on the inferior aspect of C3 (arrow). This is the result of a hyperextension injury when the anterior longitudinal injury, pulls off a fragment of bone. Note the disc degeneration with posterior osteophytosis at C5/6.

One of the main limitations of radiographs is the inability to see surrounding soft tissue structures such as the spinal cord. Visibility of the spinal cord and spinal canal can be improved by injecting contrast medium into the cerebrospinal fluid space alongside the spinal cord. This investigation, known as a myelogram (Figures 6a and 6b) is useful for demonstrating compression of the spinal cord, nerve roots and post traumatic tears in the spinal canal lining ("dura") (Figure 6c). However, it gives little information about non-expansile lesions within the spinal cord. It is less commonly performed nowadays with the advent of MRI.

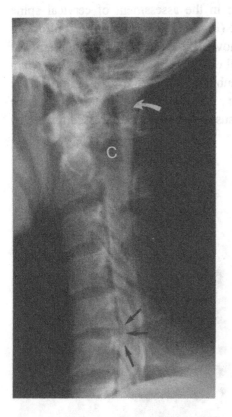 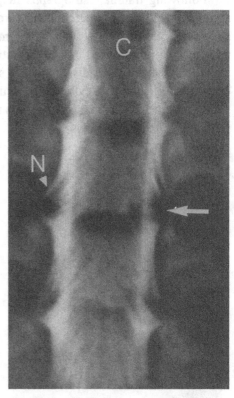

Figure 6a. Cervical myelogram lateral view. Contrast within the spinal canal (curved arrow) outlines the spinal cord (c). Note how the curvature of the cervical canal is abnormal and there is an indentation within the anterior portion of the cervical canal at C5/6 (black arrows). This indentation is the sign of a disc protusion at this level.

Figure 6b. Cervical myelogram antero-posterior view. Contrast within the spinal canal outlines the spinal cord (C) and nerve roots (N). Note how there is incomplete filling of one nerve root sheath (straight arrow) indicating compression of the nerve root at this level.

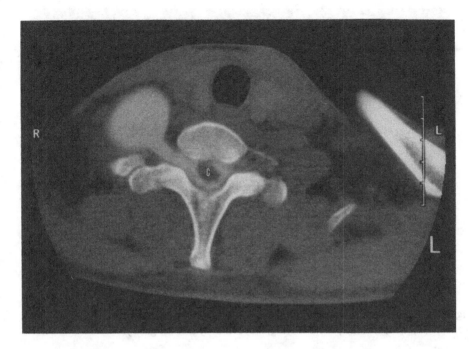

Figure 6c. CT myelogram of cervical spine in a patient with paralysis of the right arm following a motorbike accident. There is a large leak of contrast on the right side (arrow). This indicates a torn nerve root at this level which may have occurred if the arm was trapped and severely pulled. C = cervical cord.

COMPUTED TOMOGRAPHY

Computer tomography (CT) uses ionizing radiation similar to radiograph (Figure 7a). As the patient passes slowly through the scanner, thin 'slices' of the patient are examined. A computer then cleverly organises this raw data to produce complete axial images of different slices of the part examined.

CT shows cortical and trabecular detail bony better than any other imaging modality. It is excellent for examining bony injury following trauma. CT can show the extent of fractures more clearly than radiographs (Figure 7b), may demonstrate additional fractures and can show bone fragments pushed back into the spinal canal which may be compressing the spinal cord ("retropulsion") (Tehranzadeh *et al.*, 1996).

While standard CT images are obtained in the transverse (axial) plane, modern CT software allows ready reconstruction of the image data into other (sagittal, coronal, oblique) two-dimensional planes as well as three-dimensional images (Figure 7c).

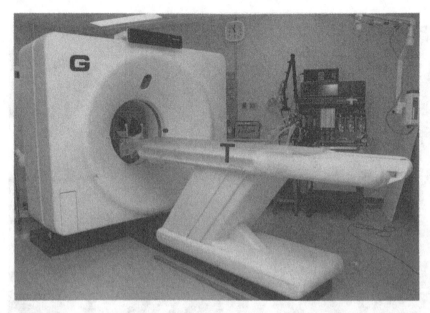

Figure 7a. CT machine. The gantry (G) houses the x-ray tube and detectors. During scanning, the table (T), on which the patient is lying, moves slowly into the gantry.

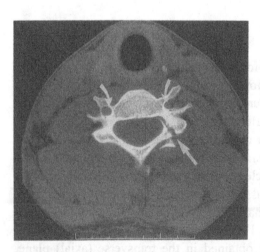

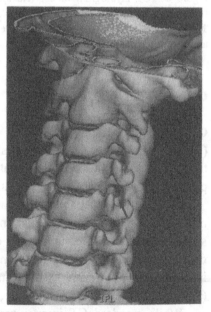

Figure 7b. Axial CT image showing a fracture of the left lamina (straight arrow). The holes (or foramen) (curved arrows) in the transverse processes contain the vertebral arteries (not seen).

Figure 7c. Three-dimensional CT reconstruction of a normal cervical spine. A neural foramen is arrowed.

Contrast medium can also be introduced into the subarachnoid space of the spinal canal via a small lumbar puncture. By slowly tilting the patient's head down, the contrast medium will collect in the cervical canal region thus helping to outline the cervical spinal cord and the nerve roots (myelogram, see above). Myelography when followed by CT is known as CT myelography. It is useful at showing traumatic avulsion of the nerve roots from the spinal cord (Figure 6c) which may occur following severe traction injury on the brachial plexus.

MAGNETIC RESONANCE IMAGING

Magnetic resonance imaging (MRI) has revolutionised imaging of the cervical spine. An MRI scanner looks like a CT machine, except that the gantry is deeper (and therefore patients may feel claustrophobic). It uses very different technology from CT. To produce an MR image, the patient is placed within the MR magnet, a radio signal is sent into the patient's body. This reacts with protons in the body tissues (though the patient does not feel anything) and a different radio signal is emitted from the patient. This signal is used to form the MR image. MR has three main advantages over CT. Firstly it can show soft tissue in better detail. Secondly, images can be obtained directly in any plane and thirdly, no radiation is involved. Many different recipes (or "sequences") are used to obtain different information about the patient's tissues. The most commonly used are T1-weighted and T2-weighted sequences. T1-weighted sequences (Figure 8a) on which fluid appears dark, are best at showing anatomy. T2-weighted sequences (Figure 8b,c) on which fluid appears bright, are best at showing pathology.

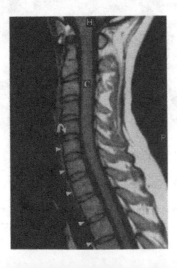

Figure 8a. Sagittal T1-weighted MR image of the cervical spine. Normal examination. Note the dark fluid (cerebrospinal fluid) surrounding the spinal cord (C), the anterior longitudinal ligament (arrowheads), the discs and the dark endplates (curved arrow) of the vertebral bodies.

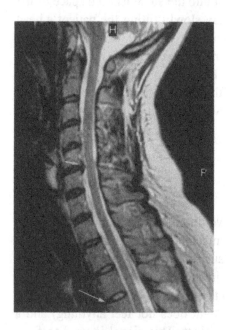

Figure 8b. T2-weighted sagittal MR image of cervical spine. Abnormal examination. A normal bright disc is shown (long arrow) in the upper dorsal region. Most of the discs in the mid- and lower cervical spine are darker as a result of degeneration. There is a disc prolapse at C5/6 (short arrow).

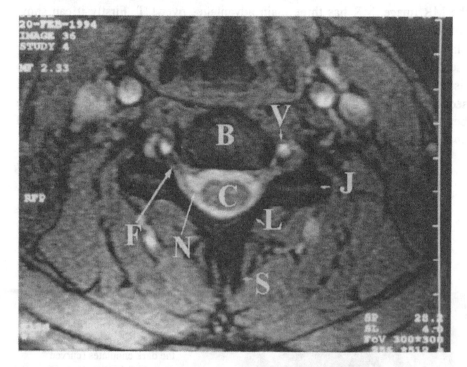

Figure 8c. T2-weighted axial MR image of cervical spine. Normal examination. C = cord. B = vertebral body, V = vertebral artery, F = neural foramen, N = nerve root, J = facet joint, L = lamina, S = spinous process.

MRI of the cervical spine is most often indicated for the assessment of degenerative disc disease and cervical radiculopathy (compression of nerve roots) and myelopathy (compression of spinal cord) (Figures 9a,b [Nagata *et al.*, 1990; Rapoport *et al.*, 1994; Tartaglino *et al.*, 1994; Rothman *et al.*, 1994]). MR can readily show disc protrusion or compression of the spinal cord or neural foramina. Chronic disc degeneration often accompanies facet joint degeneration and hypertrophy of the ligamentum flavum, all of which may be seen on an MRI. A combination of all these pathological changes (i.e. disc protrusion, ligamentum flavum hypertrophy and facet joint degeneration) will occasionally narrow the cervical canal to such a degree that the spinal cord is compressed ("spinal stenosis") (Figure 9a,b) (Rothman *et al.*, 1994).

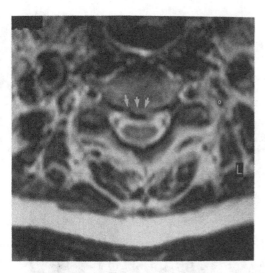
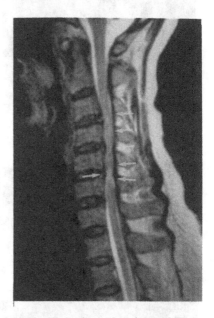

Figure 9a. Axial T2-weighted MR image showing thickening and ossification of the posterior longitudinal ligament (OPLL) (arrows) (Kameyama *et al.*, 1995).

Figure 9b. Sagittal T2-weighted MR image. In this case, the OPLL has become so severe that the spinal canal is very narrowed (stenosis). This has lead to increased cord signal intensity representing cord damage (arrows).

If the spinal cord is severely compressed it will become necrotic and fibrotic (Figure 10) (Takahashi *et al.*, 1982). MR can also readily assess any abnormalities of the craniovertebral junction (Figure 11), the vertebral bodies (Figure 12), the spinal cord or brachial plexus (Figure 13). Because MRI can obtain images in any anatomical plane, these abnormalities can be portrayed in a readily comprehensible manner.

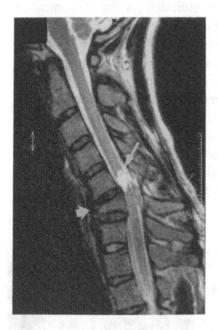

Figure 10. Sagittal T2-weighted MR image. There has been a previous anterior compression wedge fracture of C6 (short arrow) due to a hyperflexion injury. A focal area of high signal intensity is present within the cord (long arrow) representing cord damage.

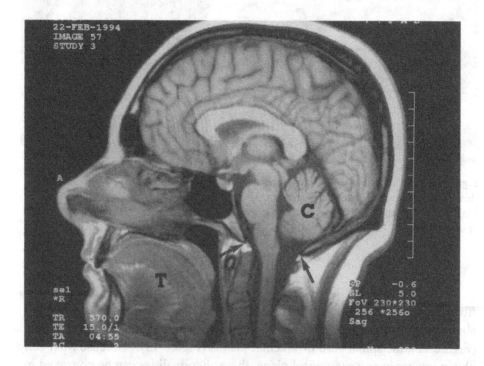

Figure 11. T1-weighted sagittal MR images showing the brain and upper spinal cord. The area between the two arrows is the foramen magnum through which passes the spinal cord. C = cerebellum.

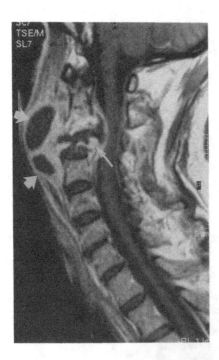

Figure 12. T1-weighted sagittal MR image of cervical spine with gadolinium enhancement. Vertebral osteomyelitis. There is severe destruction of the L3 vertebral body (long arrow) and the lower part of C2 in associated with a posterior and anterior paravertebral abscesses (short arrows). Tuberculosis was the cause.

Figure 13. Coronal T1-weighted MT image. The nerves of the brachial plexus passing from the neck to the arms are arrowed on both sides.

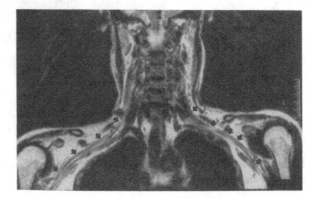

ADDITIONAL TECHNIQUES

Whilst radiographs, CT and MRI are the mainstay of cervical imaging, other investigations are more useful in certain clinical settings. For example, ultrasound scanning is very useful for examining the paravertebral soft tissues of the neck. As it can not penetrate bone, it gives no information on the bony structures or spinal canal contents. Nuclear medicine studies are much more sensitive than radiographs at showing bony metastases (Figure 14).

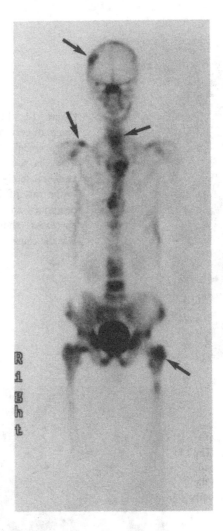

Figure 14. Isotope bone scan showing multiple "hot spots" some of which are arrowed. These represent multiple bone metastases.

CONCLUSION

Cervical spine imaging has come a long way over the past two decades. Earlier and more accurate diagnosis of cervical spine disorders is now possible. CT remains the examination method of choice for investigating cortical and trabecular bony detail, including the evaluation of spinal fractures, assessing foraminal size and ossification of the posterior longitudinal ligament whilst CT myelography is useful for assessing traumatic nerve root avulsions and dural tears. For all other disorders, MRI is the preferred examination. MRI can show ligaments, discs, vertebrae, neural foramina, spinal canal, cord and the paravertebral muscles. As a result, the natural history of many cervical spine disorders can be studied (Bush *et al.*, 1997), unnecessary operations negated and new, more appropriate treatment strategies developed.

References:

Bush K., Chaudhuri R., Hillier S., Penny J. The pathomorphologic changes that accompany the resolution of cervical radiculopathy. A prospective study with repeat magnetic resonance imaging. Spine 1997;22:183-6.

Nagata K., Kiyonaga K., Ohashi T., *et al.* Clinical value of magnetic resonance imaging for cervical myelopathy. Spine 1990;15:1088-96.

Rapoport R.J., Flanders A.E., Tartaglino L.M. Intradural extramedullary causes of myelopathy. Semin Ultrasound CT MR 1994;15:189-225.

Rothman M.I., Zoarshi G.H., Akhtar N. Extradural causes of myelopathy. Semin Ultrasound CT MR 1994;15:226-49.

Takahashi M., Yamashita Y., Sakamoto Y., Kojima R. Chronic cervical cord compression: clinical significance of increased signal intensity on MR images. Radiology 1989;172:219-24.

Tartaglino L.M., Flanders A.E., Rapoport R.J. Intramedullary causes of myelopathy. Semin Ultrasound CT MR 1994;15:158-88.

Tehranzadeh J., Palmer S. Imaging of cervical spine trauma. Semin Ultrasound CT MR 1996;17:93-104.

Suggested reading list:

Brachie-Adjei O., Squillante R.G. Tuberculosis of the spine. Orthop Clin North Am 1996;27:95-103.

Kameyama T., Hashizume Y., Ando T., *et al.* Spinal cord morphology and pathology in ossification of the posterior longitudinal ligament. Brain 1995; 118(Pt 1):263-78.

CHAPTER 7

CERVICAL SPINAL TRAUMA AND ITS SURGICAL TREATMENT

Y.L. Lee

INTRODUCTION

The goals of the treatment of cervical spine trauma are to preserve neural functions, prevent debilitating deformity and provide an optimal condition for recovery and rehabilitation. An understanding of the concepts of neurological injury and cervical instability are critical towards accomplishing these goals.

MECHANISM OF INJURY

Cervical spine trauma in Hong Kong often results from road traffic accident involving hyperextension injury of the neck. Falling from great heights is another main cause of cervical spine trauma in construction site workers. Low energy trauma such as falling from level ground, rarely induces cervical spine injury, except in the elderly or patients with rheumatoid necks. Diving sports and gunshot trauma are rare in Hong Kong, although they are relatively common in North America.

Cervical spinal trauma can be divided into injury to the vertebral column and/or the spinal cord. The muscle, ligaments and bony structures can be injured from multiple force vectors, such as flexion, extension, distraction, compression, rotation and shearing. The spinal cord will be damaged when the above structures fail to dissipate the energy of an impact. Direct force impact or indirect compression by a ruptured intervertebral disc or bony fragments may cause spinal cord injury. Occasionally, the cord can also be damaged without evidence of injury to the vertebral column. Such cord injury without radiographic abnormalities (SCIWORA) usually occurs in either very young adults or elderly patients with a background of cervical spondylosis.

MANAGEMENT

1. General principles

Patients with suspected spinal cord injury need specialised management, right from the scene of the accident. Severe neck pain, muscle spasm and paralysis of the extremities with alterations in cutaneous sensation are all typical physical signs of the injury. According to our experience, there is a high incidence of cervical spine injury associated in patients with significant head injuries. Therefore, unconscious patients should be initially treated for spinal cord or column injury. Their necks should be kept in neutral position. Gentle axial traction applied to the head will be helpful in immobilising the patient's neck during the transfer to hospital.

At the Accident and Emergency Department, a multi-disciplinary medical team consisting of trauma, neurosurgical, orthopaedic, thoracic and general surgeons, and an anesthesiologist should be on hand to evaluate the patient, because 50~60% of the patients will have various types of associated injuries. Active resuscitation and medical stabilisation of respiration and circulation are essential before any other management procedures.

Neurogenic shock must be differentiated from haemorrhagic shock in a hypotensive patient. Interrupting sympathetic outflow to the heart and peripheral vasculature can cause bradycardia and hypotension. The patient may then have a problem with the distribution of intravascular volume rather than a true hypovolemia. Consequently, vigorous fluid resuscitation can produce fatal pulmonary edema, especially in elderly patients.

2. Diagnosis

A complete neurologic examination and a properly taken plain radiograph are usually adequate in the establishment of a diagnosis. The level of lesion and whether the injury is complete or incomplete must be determined. The level of consciousness and integrity of cranial nerves, motor and sensory functions in the arms and legs should be assessed. Reflexes, including deep tendon, abdominal, cremasteric and plantar reflexes should be examined. A lateral cervical spine x-ray should be obtained and supplemented by anteroposterior and open-mouth views. All cervical vertebrate through the first thoracic vertebrae should be examined in either the "pulled-shoulder" or "swimmer's" views. Other radiological investigations like computed tomography (CT) and magnetic resonance imaging (MRI) have been discussed in more detail in the previous chapter.

3. Surgical management

(a) Principle of immobilisation

At the site of the accident, the patient should be secured to a firm board or stretcher. The neck is kept neutral using two rolled towels with a strap across the forehead. Soft cranial cervical foam is, however, preferable if available from the ambulance team.

Although the prescription of neck collar, either soft or hard type, is not necessary in acute situations, it will be recommended in case the patient has gross instability of the cervical spine. This is because the neck is supported when the collar is applied.

Cranial tongs can be easily applied as soon as cervical instability is confirmed. A few pins are inserted into the skull 1 cm above the tips of the ears in the coronal alignment with the external auditory meatus. Axial traction with a neckroll (not a sandbag) behind the neck can easily and safely be used to correct the deformity, and can even be performed by general trauma surgeons.

Halo ring application (Figure 1) is indicated when manipulation of the neck is required to reduce facet joint dislocation or fracture dislocation of the cervical spine. The ring will also be indicated if a post-operative halo vest is required to provide external immobilisation until the fracture heals. Halo ring traction should be applied only by orthopaedic specialists because 50% of patients face complications, including pin loosening, pin site infection, osteomyelitis and subdural intracranial abscess.

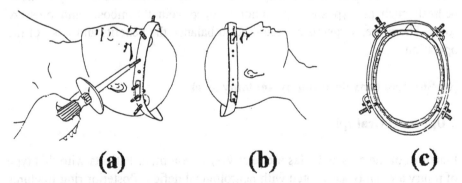

(a)   **(b)**   **(c)**

Figure 1. Halo ring immobilisation method: (a) insertion of halo ring with tonque screw driver;   (b) lateral view with ring inserted; (c) axial view with ring inserted.

Proper immobilisation of the neck is essential whenever cervical spinal cord injury is suspected. This measure should be taken to protect the neck before transfer for further investigation or to the intensive care unit. When patients only have minor fractures or soft tissue injuries without neurology deficits, they can be immobilised with various types of neck collars, including Somi brace, Philadelphia collar or soft foam.

(b) Medical treatment and timing of surgical treatment

Spinal cord injury and nerve root injury primarily result from mechanical deformation of the neural elements after fracture or dislocation. Following this primary accident, progressive biochemical, vascular and biomechanical changes can occur and lead to secondary conditions and result in necrosis or even permanent damage to neural tissues.

Many investigators have proposed that the best immediate treatment to protect the patients against developing secondary conditions is to limit the amount of irreversible neurologic injury. Currently two pharmacological agents have been shown to be beneficial to patients with spinal cord injuries and they are methylprednisolone and GM-1 ganglioside. High dosage of methylprednisolone administered within eight hours of injury has been shown to be effective in the National Spinal Cord Injury Study 2 (NASCIS 2) and GM-1 ganglioside is being investigated in a multicenter study.

The optimal time to perform surgical intervention for patients with cervical spinal disorders remain to be controversial in literature. In the case where neurological status is acutely deteriorating, early surgical decompression is preferred. However, in patients with incomplete neurology injury, there is no data to support that the surgical outcome will be better in patients with early decompression than those with late decompression. Certainly early mobilisation of patient can help to avoid the complications of prolonged bedrest, such as hypostatic pneumonia, deep vein thrombosis and pressure sores. Therefore, surgeons are required to balance the benefits and risks of the operation.

(c) Surgical consideration by anatomy level

i. Upper cervical spine

Fractures of the axis and atlas are relatively uncommon. Patients with this type of injury are rarely associated with neurological deficit. Posterior ring fractures of the atlas are usually caused by hyperextension of the occiput, thus squashing the atlas and axis. Lateral radiographs may demonstrate C1 fractures. A CT scan, however, is required to investigate the fracture pattern. A fracture of the axis can be a stable fracture provided the transverse ligament remains intacted. Healing can be successfully achieved by using a halo vest to immobilise the head and neck for 8 to 12 weeks. Rupture of the transverse ligament may cause instability at C1/2. If the lateral masses of C1 separate more than 7 mm in an anteroposterior radiograph, this may indicate that the transverse ligament is no longer intact. Posterior C1-C2 arthrodesis is then indicated. The common mechanism of C2 fracture is forcible neck hyperextension resulting from falls or motor vehicle accidents when the patient's face struck the windshield or dashboard (Figure 2). If signs and symptoms like upper cervical neck pain, persistent tenderness at C2 and soft tissue swelling greater than 5 mm anterior to C3 on a lateral radiograph are found, further investigation with CT scans is needed (Figure 3). For a fracture of the odontoid process, the degree of dens dislocation is the most determining factor for its treatment. Posterior C1-2 arthrodesis or anterior odontoid screw fixation is recommended as an initial treatment for fractures with displacement of more than 6 mm. However, most of the axis fractures can be treated successfully with halo-vest immobilisation for 10 to 12 weeks.

ii. Lower cervical spine

Acute cervical injury between C3 and T1 are more common than that in the upper cervical region. The treatment requires careful consideration and individualised therapy. Fractures of cervical vertebrate body that remain in alignment or have been reduced to anatomical alignment will heal well with external immobilisation, unless marked concomitant ligamentous disruption is present. A small percentage of patients with such injuries experience late cervical instability which is difficult to identify before primary therapy is begun. Therefore, regular follows up with these patients are necessary. When neurological impairment is found the patient can initially be treated with methylprednisolone. Anterior decompression of the spinal canal and strut graft arthrodesis with anterior plate fixation can be performed.

Some patients with unilateral or bilateral dislocated and locked facets joints can be managed non-operatively. Reduction can be achieved by halo traction and gentle manipulation in extension. Once the cervical spine is aligned, the fracture can heal with the application of halo-vest to immobilise the neck for 12 to 16 weeks. Irreducible dislocations are treated with open reduction and internal fixation. Bilateral facet dislocations are commonly associated with the disruption of posterior ligamentous elements. Therefore, posterior arthrodesis with rigid fixation is recommended.

Minor injuries often result from hyperextension, but most of them are stable. These include anterior longitudinal ligament avulsion fractures, undisplaced lateral mass fracture, laminar fractures and spinal process fractures. Stable flexion injuries usually involve body compression fracture of the vertebral body (Figures 4a and b). They are not associated with neurological injury and can be managed with immobilisation using a cervical orthosis for 8 to 12 weeks. Subsequently, flexion-extension radiographs should be taken to confirm that the healing process is proceeding well.

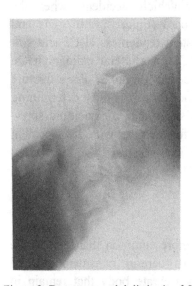

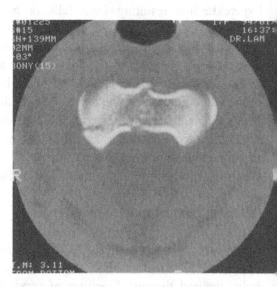

Figure 2. Fracture spondylolisthesis of C2 clearly shown in plain radiograph.

Figure 3. Fracture body of C2 with a fracture line which is only visible in CT scan.

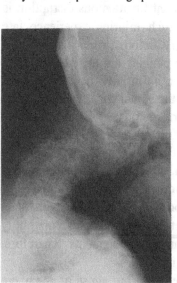

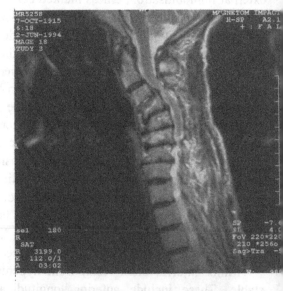

Figure 4a. Trauma film shows extensive background degenerative changes in the cervical spine.

Figure 4b. MRI film shows compressive fracture in the upper C4 level with neural tissue compression.

'WHIPLASH' INJURY

The problem of 'whiplash' and its associated disorders commonly refers to the hyperextension followed by flexion of the neck. The injury occurs to occupants of a car that is hit from behind by another vehicle. The insult may result in bony or soft tissue injuries, which in turn may lead to a variety of clinical manifestations (Whiplash-Associated Disorders WAD).

The pathophysiology is very similar to that of post-concussion syndrome. Muscle tears, haemorrhage, ligament rupture, disc avulsion, spinal and sympathetic nerve injury have all been demonstrated in various studies. The patient may exhibit a variety of symptoms at different periods of time. Complaints include neck and back pain, headache, dizziness, paraesthesia, weakness and occasionally cognitive disorder or visual impairment.

The diagnosis of WAD can usually be made clinically. Victims in motor vehicle accidents should be examined thoroughly with plain radiographs and other appropriate imaging investigation if necessary. Most cases of WAD are seldom associated with other injuries. They also tend to heal naturally. Interventions include active mobilisation, manipulation and exercise in combination with analgesics or non-steroidal anti-inflammatory agents. Symptoms can be relieved using heat, ice, laser, and transcutaneous electrical stimulation which can also help to promote early mobilisation and return to usual activities. Over dependence on neck collar or medications should be cautioned. A compassionate sympathetic approach by the clinician is important to prevent prolonged disability.

CONCLUSION

Prevention of traumatic spinal cord injury is the best measure in cervical spine trauma, since the social and economic consequence of neurological injuries are devastating. The treatment approach and timing of surgical interventions must be based on the level and severity of injury and the patient's overall medical condition. Pharmacological treatment for acute spinal cord trauma hold promise for improved sensory and motor outcomes. Advanced surgical technology and physiotherapy can help to restore maximal neck function.

Suggested reading list:

Aebi M., Zuber K., Marchesi D. Treatment of cervical spine injuries with anterior plates: Indications, techniques and results. Spine 1991;16:S38-45.

Bohlman H.H. Acute fracture and dislocations of the cervical spine: An analysis of 300 hospitalized patients and review of the literature. J Bone Joint Surg 1979;61A:1119-42.

Brachen M.B., Shepard M.J., Collins W.F. *et al*. A randomized, controlled trial of methylprednisolone or naloxone in the treatment of acute spinal cord injury: Results of the second national acute spinal cord injury study. N Eng J Med 1990;322:1405-11.

Garfin S., Bottle M.J., Waters R.L. *et al*. Complications in the use of the halo fixation device. J Bone Joint Surg 1986;68A:320-5.

Geisler F.H., Dorsey F.C., Coleman W.P. Recovery of motor function after spinal cord injury ~ A randomized, placebo-controlled trial with gm-1 ganglioside. N Eng J Med 1991;324:1829-38.

Gunzburg R., Szpalski M. Whiplash Injuries-Current concepts in prevention, diagnosis, treatment of the cervical whiplash syndrome. Lippincott-Raven, 1998.

Pang D., Wilberger J.E. Jr. Spinal cord injury without radiographic abnormalities in children. J Neurosurg 1982;57:114-29.

CHAPTER 8

ORTHOSES FOR CERVICAL SPINAL DISORDERS

M.S. Wong

INTRODUCTION

An appropriate prescription and application of cervical orthosis require good understanding of the pathology and pathophysiology of the cervical disorder, detailed clinical assessment of the patient and accurate anticipation of the positive and negative effects of the prescribed orthosis. The cervical spine is comparatively difficult to control because it is the most mobile region of the entire spine. Therefore, the properties, functions and effects of different cervical orthoses should be understood thoroughly before any effective orthotic treatment can be provided.

In the past, the knowledge about the underlying pathology and pathophysiology of cervical spine and its supporting mechanisms were frequently ambiguous, even if the symptoms were manifested. Thus, a complete analysis on the effectiveness of an orthosis would be difficult to perform. In recent years, the biomechanics of the spine have been well outlined by some renowned fellows such as Panjabi and White (1993). Given with the sound biomechanical principles, the development of appropriate cervical orthoses can be healthy supported and the enhancement of effectiveness of orthotic management can be positively achieved.

The prescription of a cervical orthosis should include a suitably detailed description of the orthosis, instead of a series of generalised instructions, which may not match with the physician's intention or meet the individual patient's need. A mutually accepted prescription and treatment protocol among the prosthetist-orthotist, prescribing clinician and relevant therapists should be encouraged. Thus, a holistic approach of patient care can then be accomplished.

CERVICAL ORTHOSES

In 1993, with the collaboration among the International Standard Organisation (ISO), the American Academy of Orthopaedic Surgeons (AAOS), the American Academy of Orthotists and Prosthetists (AAOP), the American Orthotic and Prosthetic Association (AOPA) and the International Society for Prosthetics and Orthotics (ISPO), a commonly accepted terminology system for prosthetics and orthotics was worked out (Schuch & Pritham 1993). For cervical orthoses and their abbreviations (Redford & Patel 1995, Harris 1986), they are as follows:

      Cervical Orthosis (CO)
      Cervicothoracic Orthosis (CTO)
      Cervicothoracolumbosacral Orthosis (CTLSO)

For cervical orthoses, there are basically two types of cervical orthoses, the prefabricated (off-the-shelf) orthoses and the custom-made orthoses (Berger et al. 1983). In the prefabricated cervical orthoses, they include two basic types, neck collars and post appliances, while the custom-made orthoses have a large variety of designs. The function of some cervical orthoses is mainly aimed at reminding the users to restrict their head and neck motions, while some other orthoses can apply forces to position or immobilise the head, to limit the motion of the head and neck, and/or reduce the load on the cervical spine. The level of cervical orthoses in controlling neck motion varies greatly. For example, a soft collar can render only mild control, while the halo-type orthosis can offer effective constraint in all directions of motion. A good understanding of the properties of different orthoses is therefore important (Sandler *et al.* 1996). The immobilisation capability of some common cervical orthoses is proposed in Table 1.

Table 1. Comparison of the immobilisation capability of the common cervical orthoses.

Cervical Orthoses	Flexion	Extension	Lateral Flexion	Rotation	Axial Unloading
Basic Neck Collar	** / ***	* / **	* / **	* / **	*
Philadelphia Collar	** / ***	**	**	**	*
Post Orthosis	***	***	*/**	**	#
SOMI	***	**	**	**	#
Cuirass or Minerva Orthosis	***	***	***	***	#
Halo Orthosis	***	***	***	***	#

* mild control, ** moderate control, *** sufficient control, # variable axial unloading

PRE-FABRICATED CERVICAL ORTHOSES

1. Basic Collars: Soft Collar and Rigid Collar
(Flexion-extension control orthoses)

Collars are orthoses that embrace the neck region (Figure 1 and Figure 2). Some designs are with height adjustment. They are either single or multiple layered with variable firmness. The materials used may include spongy rubber, resilient polyethylene foam, felt and rigid polyethylene sheeting.

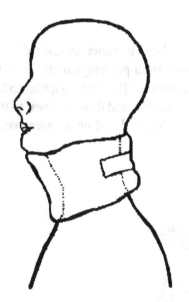

Figure 1. Soft neck collar.

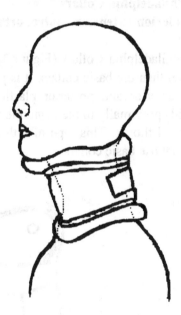

Figure 2. Rigid neck collar.

Functions

They can only satisfy mild to moderate control of flexion and extension, but a relatively minimal constraint to lateral flexion and rotation. It can also act as a reminder for the users to limit their head and neck motions through sensory feedback, and to retain body heat, which may help to promote soft tissue healing and decrease muscle spasm.

Suggestions and Considerations

They are usually applied for degenerative changes or soft tissue injuries. It is known that the cervical foraminae close down in extension and open up in flexion. The posterior part of collar should be made high enough under the occiput to resist or prevent extension or hyperextension. For greater control, a mandibular reinforcement may be added to form a more rigid collar. Prefabricated collars are sometimes difficult to fit comfortably due to a mismatch of contours between the orthosis and the patient's neck. Such problems can be solved using a custom-made collar. Johnson *et al.* (1977) studied several cervical orthoses and reported that soft collars can reduce neck motion in the sagittal plane by 26%. It basically cannot limit rotation or lateral bending.

2. Philadelphia Collars
(Flexion-extension control orthoses)

The Philadelphia Collars (Figure 3) provide relatively better control of neck motion than the basic collars. It is prefabricated from polyethylene foam, with rigid anterior and posterior plastic reinforcements. The Philadelphia collar extends proximally to the mandible and at the occiput, and distally down to the proximal thorax. This type of orthosis covers the head and neck extensively, unlike those basic collars.

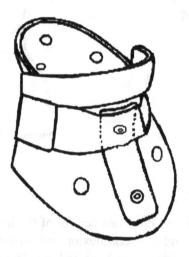

Figure 3. Philadelphia Collar.

Functions

It can restrict neck motion and retain heat. The anterior and posterior plastic reinforcements give this orthosis greater control to cervical flexion, extension, rotation and lateral bending than those provided by soft collars. The anterior and posterior plastic reinforcements also allow selective positioning of the head on the sagittal plane.

3. Post Orthoses
(Flexion-extension-lateral-rotary control orthoses)

The Post Orthosis is divided into the anterior part and posterior part. The anterior part consists of a sternal plate, a mandibular support and one or two uprights while the posterior part consists of an interscapular plate, an occipital support and one or two posts. The anterior and posterior parts are usually connected by head straps between the mandibular and occipital supports and by the shoulder straps between the interscapular and sternal plates (Figure 4). The height of the posts is adjustable and the angulation of the plates can also be changed by means of the swivel joints between the posts and the plates. This type of orthosis is usually prefabricated from aluminium and fitted with soft padding for enhancing fitness and comfort. The four-post orthosis gives better control in restricting the lateral motion of the neck, although it is slightly cumbersome than the one with two posts.

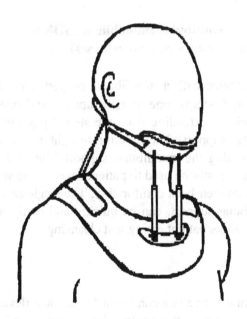

Figure 4. Post Orthosis.

Functions

They can provide control for flexion and extension of the head and cervical spine by the forces applied from the mandibular and occipital supports. The lateral flexion and rotation can also be limited by the orthoses. Altering the length of the posts can modify the head weight on the cervical spine.

Suggestions and Considerations

The motion control can be increased by a rigid attachment between the mandibular and occipital supports, and by enlarging the contact area of the two supports. Some Post Orthoses may extend to the mid-thoracic region that can further increase the immobilisation not only for cervical flexion and extension but also limiting some thoracic flexion and extension as well. These orthoses are classified as cervicothoracic flexion-extension control orthoses. A rigid collar with the mandibular and occipital supports may be necessary if the patient cannot tolerate the Post Orthosis.

In Johnson's study (1977), a four-poster was found to allow 21% flexion and extension, 27% rotation and 4% lateral bending. As compared with the Philadelphia collar, this design provides relatively good control of head motion. The indications for two-post and four-post CTOs are the same as those of the head-cervical orthoses. However, post orthoses can not keep warmth as done by the Philadelphia collars.

4. Sterno-occipital-mandibular-immobiliser, SOMI (Flexion-extension-rotary control orthoses)

This orthosis is a device with a mandibular support, an occipital support, a sternal plate, two back straps, one anterior upright and two lateral uprights. The two lateral uprights extending from the sternal plate for maintaining the position of occipital support. The anterior upright raises anteriorly from a sternal plate for locating the mandibular support (Figure 5). Because of the design, the SOMI can easily be used to patients even in the supine position and permits them to lie on their back comfortably. The single anterior upright, with its attached mandibular support, can be quickly and easily removed from the sternal plate. It can allow patient eating and cleansing.

Functions

The SOMI gives almost the same constraint for cervical flexion and rotation as the Post Orthoses, however, the control for extension and lateral flexion is relatively lesser.

Suggestions and Considerations

Using a prefabricated polyethylene shell and a Dacron head strap, the SOMI can be modified for replacing the mandibular support. This strap allows the patient free for eating and provides some degree of flexion control as it surrounds the forehead and fastens to the occipital support (Figure 6). It is for temporary use but not for a definitive treatment.

Johnson *et al.* (1977) studied the functions of SOMIs and their results showed that 28% flexion and extension, 34% rotation and 66% lateral bending were recorded as compared to the normal range of motion. It means that their effectiveness is comparable to the Post Orthoses.

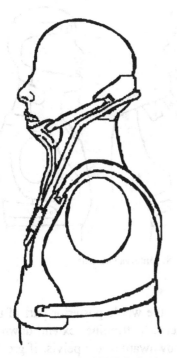

Figure 5. Basic SOMI Orthosis.

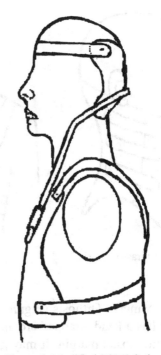

Figure 6. Modified SOMI Orthosis

CUSTOM-MADE ORTHOSES

Custom-made orthoses are specially designed to render better control of neck motion in all directions. They can also restrict thoracic motion to various degrees, depending on the amount of downward extension to the thorax. Orthoses extending distally beyond the upper thorax are classified as cervicothoracic orthoses, CTOs. These custom-molded orthoses can be either made of high-temperature thermoplastics (e.g. polyethylene) molded on the patient's plaster model or low-temperature thermoplastics (e.g. synergy) directly formed on the patient.

1. Cuirass and Minerva Orthoses

The upper trimlines of Cuirass Orthosis (Figure 7) go proximally to the chin, mandible and occiput. Its lower trimlines terminate at about 2.5 cm above the inferior angles of the scapulae. Subjected to the level of control, it may further extend downward to the inferior costal margin.

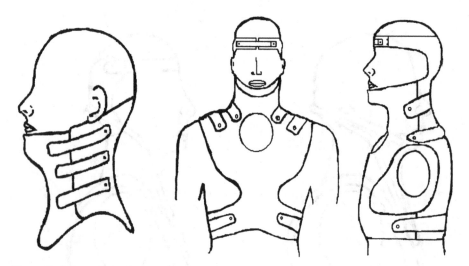

Figure 7. Cuirass Orthosis.   Figure 8. Minerva Orthosis.

The Minerva Orthosis (Figure 8) encircles the whole posterior part of the skull. It has a band wrapped around the forehead. Its trimlines extend down to the inferior costal margin. It may go further downward to the pelvis, if greater controls over cervical and thoracic motion are required.

Functions

These two types of orthosis provide immobilising forces under the chin and occiput, which can limit flexion and extension, lateral motion and rotation of the neck. It can also locate the head in a particular position and reduce the load on the cervical spine from the head. Various degrees of thoracic motion can be also constrained.

2. Halo Orthosis

The Halo Orthosis (Figure 9) renders the greatest control of cervical spinal motion as compared with other cervical orthoses. There are several designs and its basic components normally include a halo-ring, distraction rods, shoulder bars and a distal fixation component. The halo-ring encircles the skull at the location just above the eyebrow and is fixed in place by four metal pins that insert a few millimetres deep into the skull. Distraction rods are then attached to the halo ring and to the shoulder bars, which are further attached to a distal fixation component. It can be a vest, a body jacket, a pelvic girdle, a pelvic loop or femoral transfixing pins.

Functions

Using a Halo Orthosis, the head is rigidly fixed upon the thorax. The distraction forces provided by the orthosis can be used to immobilise head and decrease the head loading on the cervical spine for facilitating the healing process.

Suggestions and Considerations

Johnson *et al.* (1977) found that Halo Orthosis allows 4% cervical flexion and extension, 1% rotation and 4% lateral bending. Wang *et al.* (1988) investigated the effectiveness of vest length of the Halo Orthosis in stabilising the cervical spine. They reported that a lesion at the upper cervical spine could be treated effectively by Halo Orthosis only with a half-length vest. However, if the lesion is below C4, extension of the vest length down to the 12th rib is required to provide adequate stability.

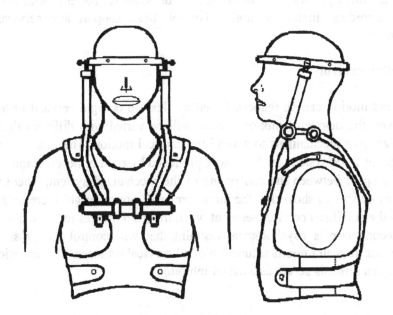

Figure 9. Halo Orthosis

Benzel *et al.* (1989) compared the immobilisation capability between the Minerva Orthosis and a Halo Orthosis in 10 ambulatory patients with unstable cervical spines. They found that intervertebral motion in the sagittal plane was reduced at each level with the Minerva Orthosis. The average segmental movement allowed at each level was 2.3° with a Minerva Orthosis and 3.7° with a Halo Orthosis, except for the Cl-C2 segment. They concluded that the Minerva Orthosis provided better immobilisation power than that of the Halo Orthosis.

Patients may also feel that the Minerva Orthosis is more comfortable than the Halo Orthosis. Maiman *et al.* (1989) investigated the immobilisation effect of thermoplastic Minerva Orthosis. They found that the degree of limitation in the sagittal motion was equal to that given by a Halo Orthosis, except between occiput-C1, C3-4 and C6-7. These results have reconfirmed the findings of the report of Millington *et al.* (1987). Maiman *et al.* (1989) have suggested that Minerva Orthosis is better than Halo Orthosis because it is comfortable to wear on the neck and the application procedure is easy which will further encourage patients to participate in the rehabilitation program.

EFFECTS OF CERVICAL ORTHOSES

Positive Effects

There are three positive effects of cervical orthoses for patients with cervical spinal disorders, including motion control, head support and cervical re-alignment.

1. Motion control

The head motion can be reduced by either flexible or rigid cervical orthoses. However, the degree of motion control will be varied with different designs. There are two mechanisms to control the cervical motion. The first one is the three-point force system, such as those produced by rigid orthoses, stabilise the cervical spine between the end points of the mechanical system. There were some evidences to show that the intersegmental motion might increase at the end of the stabilised cervical segment when the trunk moves in some orthoses. The second one is psychological restraint that will control the gross head movement. It is an important function of all cervical orthoses. The sensation of wearing an orthosis serves as a useful inhibitor.

2. Head support

The head support can be achieved by the application of either the axial traction and/or the three-point force system. Morris (1961) demonstrated that the axial traction could effectively reduce the load of the cervical spine through the chin and occipital supports of the cervical orthosis. The three-point force system to support the head is relatively less important because once the head is vertically positioned, the weight of the head will be transmitted to the thorax mainly through the cervical spine, rather than the orthosis.

3. Cervical realignment

The realignment of the cervical spine is achieved by the three-point force systems, which stimulate muscles to withdraw from uncomfortable pressure points. This can produce shift of gravitational forces away from diseased body parts. For example, extension of the head will produce weight transfer from the vertebral bodies to the posterior elements of the cervical spine. Similarly, flexion will shift the load from the posterior elements of the cervical spine to the vertebral bodies and anterior intervertebral discs (Norton & Brown 1957).

Negative Effects

Besides the positive effects, it is even more important to know the negative effects in the application of cervical orthoses.

1. Joint tightness and/or contracture

It is known that immobilisation of the cervical spine may cause cervical stiffness. Fibrosis may then result and healing will be retarded. In order to avoid this, rehabilitation program should be started when the patient's condition is allowed, instead of some weeks or months later.

2. Muscular weakness and/or atrophy

The restriction of cervical motion will decrease the muscular activities of the neck. Although this can reduce symptoms and promote healing, it may also induce muscular weakness or atrophy. Once the treatment is discontinued, the patient may be thus vulnerable to episode of the same disease. Therefore, this consequence must be avoided. Gradual discontinuation or weaning off for the orthosis should be encouraged as soon as the symptom becomes improved. An appropriate exercise regimen should be implemented when the patient's condition is allowed.

3. Psychological conviction

Berger *et al.* (1983) pointed out that because of the emotional disorders often lie beneath the surface of the personality, the psychological conviction that may follow and enhance physical dependence. The neurotic behavior may develop quickly after injury and psychotic patterns may even emerge. Such problems must be considered at the onset of therapy, or they may soon go beyond the original disease. These emotional problems would be enhanced by overtreatment; therefore, any treatment modality must be clearly re-evaluated before it further somatizes emotional symptom complexes.

4. Irritation of other symptoms

Waters and Morris (1970) have demonstrated an increased electromyographic activity of trunk muscles during rapid ambulation when an orthosis was worn. This is assumed due to restraint of normal motions, which occur during gait and consequently increased demands on the other spinal musculature to stabilize the spine. Thus, the orthosis itself may create some adverse effects. Some cervical orthoses, by decreasing motion within the boundaries of their mechanical systems, may cause increased motion at the ends of the restrained segments. If disease is present in this end region, symptoms may be increased.

CONCLUSION

Whenever an orthosis is prescribed, the specific orthotic functions required by individual patient as well as the positive and negative effects should be well covered and anticipated accordingly. Further clinical studies are definitely required to evaluate the effectiveness and possible effects of different cervical orthoses. This can only be accomplished by underpinning with the team approach spirit through sharing of clinical experiences, running biomechanical studies and conducting outcome evaluation.

References:

Benzel E.C., Hadden T.A., Saulsbery C.M. A comparison of the Minerva and Halo jackets for stabilisation of the cervical spine. J Neurosurg 1989;70:411-4.

Berger N., Edelstein J., Fishman S., Krebs D., Springer W. Spinal Orthotics. New York University 1983:37-48.

Harris J.D. Cervical Orthoses. Third edition. In: Redford J.B. ed, Orthotics Etc, Baltimore, Williams & Wilkins, 1986:100-21.

Johnson R.M., Hart D.L., Simmons E.F. *et al.* Cervical Orthoses. J Bone Joint Surg 1977;59A:330-2.

Maiman D., Millington P., Novak S. *et al.* The effect of the thermoplastic Minerva body jacket on cervical spine motion. J Neurosurg 1989;25: 363-8.

Millington P.J., Ellingsen J.M. Thermoplastic Minerva body jacket - a practical alternative to current methods of cervical spine stabilisation: A clinical report". Phys Ther 1987;67:223-5.

Morris J., Lucas D., Bressler B. Role of the trunk in the stability of the spine. J Bone Joint Surg 1961;43A:327-51.

Norton P., Brown T. The immobilisation efficiency of back braces. J Bone Joint Surg 1957;39A:111-39.

Panjabi M.M., Vasavada A., White A.A. Cervical spine biomechanics. Semin Spine Surg 1993;5:10-61.

Redford J.B., Patel A.T. State of the art reviews. Spine 1995;9:673-88.

Sandler A.J., Dvorak J., Humke T., Grob D., Daniels W. The effectiveness of various cervical orthoses. Spine 1996;21:1624-29.

Schuch C.M., Pritham C.H. International standards organisation terminology. J Prosthetics and Orthotics 1993;6:29-33.

Wang G.J., Moskal J.T., Albert T. *et al.* The effect of halo vest length on stability of the cervical spine. J Bone Joint Surg 1988;70A:357-60.

Waters R.L., Morris J.M. Effect of spinal supports on the electrical activity of muscles of the trunk. J Bone Joint Surg 1970;52A:51-60.

PART III

Occupational and Sports Injuries of the Neck

CHAPTER 9

OCCUPATIONAL DISORDERS OF THE NECK

Bosco Tak Wai Chan

INTRODUCTION

Occupational cervical disorder is a collective term for musculoskeletal problems in the cervical region, which are closely associated with risk factors in the workplace. Although these disorders are termed as "injury", the causative mechanisms and pathologies are somewhat different from those of trauma. In this chapter, the nature of the occupational overuse syndrome and occupational cervical disorders are reviewed. In order to prepare ourselves to provide therapeutic interventions for these patients and prescribe preventive measures to those who are at risk of occupational disorders, it is important to understand the development of the disorders and be able to identify the risk factors in the workplace. Some effective preventive strategies for these disorders (and guidelines for proper usage of computers) will be discussed.

OCCUPATIONAL OVERUSE SYNDOME

Occupational overuse syndrome (OOS) is also known as repetitive strain injury (RSI), cumulative trauma disorder (CTD), repetitive movement injury (RMI), and work-related musculoskeletal disorders (WRMD) (Richardson & Eastlake, 1994). Different connotations are developed and used in different countries as shown in Table 1 below.

Table 1. Descriptive terms for upper limb occupational disorders in different countries.

Terms	Abbreviations	Countries
Repetitive strain injury	RSI	Australia
Repetitive motion injury	RMI	Canada
Cumulative trauma disorder	CTD	United States
Occupational cervicobranchial disorder	OCD	Sweden, Japan
Occupational overuse disorder	OOD	Australia

What is OOS?

OOS may be regarded as a health-related problem arising from an individual working beyond his/her physical capacity in the workplace. Such a simplified view provides some superficial descriptions of the problem. The National Occupational Health and Safety Committee (NOHSC) defines OOS as a term denoting a collection of conditions characterised by recurrent or persistent pain in musculo-tendinous structures, with or without physical manifestations. It may be aggravated or caused by work and is usually associated with repetitive movement and/or sustained, constrained postures and/or forceful movement. Psychological factors are also regarded as having predisposing value (NOHSC, 1989). Therefore, OOS is not a diagnosis but a grab bag term covering many causes and manifestations. In other words, it refers to a spectrum of musculoskeletal conditions ranging from poorly defined disorders to distinct medical conditions.

Some of the better recognised conditions include tenosynovitis, peritendinitis, epicondylitis, bicipital tendinitis, ulnar nerve entrapment, rotator cuff's syndrome, carpal tunnel syndrome, deQuervain's syndrome, thoracic outlet syndrome, etc. In many cases, both the distinct and the less well-defined disorders are found to co-exist (Putz-Anderson, 1992). It is interesting to know that some of the conditions were classified as trade-related disorders in the earlier days. With the advancement of medical sciences and better understanding of the nature of the disorders, the conditions are re-classified by a more anatomical way. Table 2 below shows some of the reclassified terms (Ranney, 1997).

Table 2. Reclassification of some of the terminology relates to work related disorders.

Old terms	Reclassified terms
Seamstress's cramp	Carpal tunnel syndrome
Gold polisher's hand	Ulnar nerve entrapment
Granite cutter's cramp	Vibration induced neuropathy
Stenographer hand	Carpal tunnel syndrome
Hammerer's cramp	Ulnar artery obstruction
Housemaid's knee	Patellar bursitis

OOS develops slowly and can affect many parts of the body. Many symptoms may come and then result in aching, tenderness, swelling, pain, cracking, tingling, numbness, loss of strength, loss of joint movement and diminishing coordination of the injured area. OOS is a collection of the musculoskeletal problems discussed above, it may comprise a number of specific and non-specific disorders. Therefore, the clinical presentation of a particular case will depend on the nature of its pertaining disorders.

Prevalence of OOS

Bureau of Labour Statistics (BLS) (BLS 1995) revealed that there was an extraordinary rise in work related CTD in the United States and it increased from 22,600 cases in 1981 to 332,000 cases in 1994 (Table 3). These figures suggest that CTD is a prevailing and fast-spreading condition which should receive immediate attention in order to tackle the problems and find possible solutions to them.

Table 3. Bureau of Labour statistics: data on cases due to repeated trauma from 1981 to 1994.

Year	Number of cases due to repeated trauma	Percentage of all occupational illness
1981	22,600	18
1989	146,900	52
1991	223,600	61
1993	302,400	64
1994	332,000	65

Impacts of OOS

OOS threatens to inflict individuals with illness and overwhelms corporations with increasing medical costs and lost productivity. Worker compensation claims for the disorders, such as low back strain, carpal tunnel syndrome and tendinitis, have become epidemic in today's workplace. The trend is spreading rapidly, with these disorders now representing the majority of claims and costs for worker compensation. Direct and indirect costs are estimated to exceed $100 billion annually (HSE, 1990) in the UK!

OCCUPATIONAL CERVICAL DISORDERS (OCD)

What is occupational cervical disorders?

Occupational cervical disorders (OCD) is a subgroup of OOS in which the clinical presentation and the causative factors are the same as those of OOS.

However, the problems arise in the cervical region. The Japan Association of Industrial Health proposes that the term OCD should collectively describe a wide range of work-related symptoms in the neck and upper limb (Maeda, 1982). Apart from neck and shoulder dysfunctions, OCD is characterised by symptoms such as dullness in the arms and hands, headache, general fatigue and irritability. When symptoms manifested, OCD can be separately classified into thoracic outlet syndrome, cervical disc herniation and cervical osteoarthritis according to its pathology. Tension Neck Syndrome (TNS) is one of the common form of OCD which is characterised by neck pain, a feeling of fatigue or stiffness in the neck, headache radiating from the neck, muscle tightness, palpable hardening and tender spots in muscles and straightening of the cervical spine (Ranney, 1997).

Physiological aspects

The plausible biologic mechanisms of the causation by the risk factors have been proposed to cause OOS. OOS are found in workers who frequently engage in jobs involving awkward postures, large force and highly repetitive movements. The development of OOS may result from repeated performance of work tasks over a prolonged period of time, causing repeated damage to tissue in muscles, tendons, joints, or nerve structures (Putz-Anderson, 1992). If neck muscles contract for long time during work, blood flow to the muscles is reduced. As a result, the biochemical by-products (waste substances produced by the muscles) cannot be removed quickly enough. Accumulation of these substances may then cause muscle irritation, injury and pain.

If neck muscles are not allowed to rest and recuperate, they will not be able to recover before new damage occurs. Long lasting or permanent injury will then develop with repetitive uses of the muscles. As there is repetitive forceful movements in the joints, the normal smooth cartilage becomes pitted and frayed. Eventually, segments of the cartilage may be damaged. At a later stage, the bony outgrowth of the damaged bony structure may impair joint movement and cause severe pain. These changes mark the development of degenerative joint disease or osteoarthritis.

With repetitive motions and awkward postures, the tissue surrounding the nerves become swollen which will squeeze or compress nerves and cause pain (Richardson and Eastlake, 1994). Existing injury is another important factor in determining the outcome of OOS. With repetitive motion, injured tissues become inflamed. The increase in osmotic pressure of the injured tissue will further limit circulation to the muscle. As the muscle gets damaged, its neighbour muscle groups become tensed up which will further restrict blood flow in the muscle. A vicious cycle is then set up.

Awkward posture of the neck

Taking deskwork as an example of neck flexion and protrusion, as the body inclines forward, the centre of gravity of the head is offset from the supporting line of the spine. The neck muscles have to contract harder than in neutral position in order to hold the head in position. This static contraction continuously pulls at the tendons of the neck and compresses the cervical joints. Blood flow to the neck muscles will then decrease. Metabolic wastes built up in the muscle are inadequately flushed away. Neck tissues are irritated and cause inflammation and pain. Pain in turn may lead to reflective muscle spasm, continuing the vicious cycle again. If the cycle persists, these musculoskeletal problems may precipitate and cause chronic disorders. Cervical extension will narrow the space of the intervertebral foramen. Spinal nerves or vessels may be compressed if this posture is sustained for too long or is performed repeatedly and frequently. This may provoke pain in the neck. It has been reported that hyperextension and rotation of the head will decrease the blood flow of the vertebral or carotid vessels. Symptoms of vertebral artery insufficiency will appear in these cases. (Okawara & Nibbelink, 1974).

RISK FACTORS

OCD is caused by many factors and can be divided into three main areas, job-related risk factors, personal risk factors and environmental factors. These factors can be precipitated by poor work organisation (HSE, 1990).

Job-related risk factors

Evidence shows that work exposures are associated with the development of injury. Certain work exposures pose relatively high risk. The generic attributes of work (ILO,1982) that contribute to the OCD development are as follows:
i.   Repetition
    Work activities which are done at a high rate of repetition.
ii. Force
    Work activities which require the use of excessive muscle force for a long time.
iii. Posture
    Work activities which require a fixed awkward posture for a long time (Figure 1).

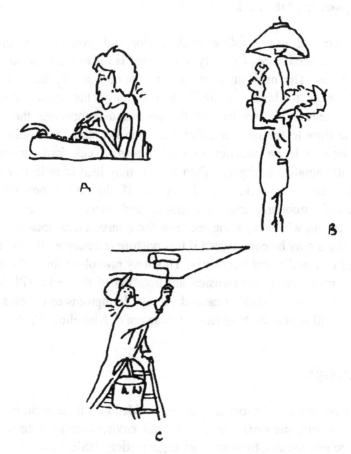

Figure 1. Poor working postures due to the physical demand of the jobs.

Putz-Anderson (1992) reconfirmed that musculoskeletal disorders of the neck and upper limbs had been frequently found in workers whose jobs involved high repetitive movements, large force and awkward postures. These can be due to non-neutral postures, extreme postures, forceful exertions, constrained or static postures, repetitive work and work that requires one to stretch beyond the shoulder height.

Table 4 shows the possible tissue changes and health outcomes associated with the risk factors discussed above. (Ranney, 1997). Shoulder-neck disorders are common in those who have to maintain a working posture with elevated arms, repetitive shoulder muscle contractions and backward head bending e.g. subcontractor. As the head of an average adult weighs 20 pounds, this posture places heavy load on the neck and shoulder.

Table 4. Possible effects of the risk factors.

Risk factor present at work	Possible tissue changes	Health outcomes
Extreme posture	Compression of blood vessels or nerves	Vertebral artery insufficiency
Static posture	Static contraction of muscles	Myalgia / Tension neck syndrome
Overhead work	Increased intramuscular pressure in supraspinatus with reduction in blood flow	Myalgia of trapezius
Forceful exertion	Strain in tendons or muscles	Muscle strain

Personal risk factors

Personal risk factors are the characteristics of workers that may affect the probability that he/she will develop OCD (Johansson & Rubenowitz, 1994; Linton & Kanwendo, 1988). These factors include:

i. Anthropometry factor
    Workspace and equipment are usually designed only for particular body sizes. Undue physical stress will be imposed upon workers with extreme body sizes.
ii. Psychological factor
    It has been suggested that the psychological factor plays an important role.
iii. Other factors
    Gender, strength, medical history, smoking habits are also suggested to be related to the occurrence of OCD.

Environmental factors

Environmental factors are characteristics of external surrounding that may affect the probabilities of workers to develop OCD (Dimberg *et al.*, 1989). For example,

i. Incorrect lighting installation may cause computer operators to adopt awkward postures to avoid shadows,
ii. Flicking light will cause stress to worker and,
iii. High noise levels may cause mental stress.

Work organisation

The following work organisation characteristics can intensify the risk factors of musculoskeletal disorders (Bergqvist *et al.*, 1995).

i. Inadequate work recovery cycles

Short recovery periods from work may not allow enough time between exertions. This will contribute to fatigue and over-exertion.

ii. Excessive working duration

Excessive working hours, such as overtime and long evening shifts, may increase the risk factors at work and decrease resting time.

iii. Unfamiliar work

New muscle groups will be recruited to perform unfamiliar job. This may cause muscle soreness.

iv. Lack of task variability

Monotonous work may increase mechanical load on a particular part of the body due to lack of postural changes. Lack of task variability will increase repetitive movements, which may increase the risk of OCD.

v. No control over work pace

Salvendy and Smith (1981) revealed that pace can amplify the development of unwanted physical and mental effects, particularly under supervision.

As a quick reference, the list below summarises the findings of common risk factors of OCD (Yu & Wong, 1996; Viikara-Juntwa *et al.*, 1994),

1. Inappropriate ergonomic workstation set-up,
2. Visual Display Unit (VDT) induced near-vision stress,
3. Asymmetrical task performance,
4. Restricted body movements,
5. Physically demanding work,
6. Repetitive movements demanding precision,
7. Work requiring that arms are raised,
8. Absence of brief (1~2 seconds) regenerative breaks during work activity,
9. Dysponesis during task performance (co-contraction, lack of inhibition of antagonist during movement),
10. Lack of somatic awareness of tension and relaxation,
11. Monotonous work position.

WHO ARE AT RISK?

Based on the above analysis, it is expected that the risk of OCD will be relatively high in those jobs which required long periods of sitting or standing and repeated movements. Dentists, subcontractors, keyboard operators, manufacturing workers, maintenance workers and fruit pickers have been identified to be at high risk of OCD because workers are frequently required to maintain an awkward and sustained posture at work and require highly repetitive work without variability (Kamwendo *et al.*, 1991).

Epidemiological context of OCD associated with work

Epidemiological studies are commonly used to investigate the risk factors associated with OCD. Sakakibara *et al.* (1995) investigated the relation between working posture and the complaints of farmers who cultivated pears and apples. They found that pear farmers were required to raise their arms and bend their head backwards more than apple farmers in picking and bagging the fruits. They also found that the prevalence of pain and stiffness in the neck, shoulders and arms was significantly higher in pear farmers than apple farmers. Symptoms of vertebral artery insufficiency were reported in some cases as well. These results suggested that the working postures of elevated arms and head tilted backwards may cause symptoms in the neck, shoulders and arms.

In a study performed by McPhee (1990), keyboard operators were found to have the highest risk factor among the other professions. Keyboard operators were nearly two and half times more likely to develop symptoms in the neck and or upper extremities than non-keyboard operators. Blader (1991) studied the occurrence of neck-shoulder problems in sewing-machine operators (SMO). They found that the incident rate of the problem was 75% in the last 12 months and 51% in the last 7 days of the study. Reports of daily neck and shoulder discomfort was 26%. Moreover, 27% and 37% of the operators had problems leading to limited working time and leisure time respectively. TNS was the most frequent complaints in the operators, followed by cervical syndrome. Prolonged static load in the neck and shoulder was suggested to be the cause of the neck-shoulder problems in the SMO. Holmstrom *et al.* (1992) studied the prevalence rate of neck and shoulder disorders in a randomly selected sample of 1773 construction workers. The 1-year incident rate of neck and shoulder disorders was 56% and pain in the neck or shoulder was 12%.

Yu *et al.* (1993) performed a telephone interview to explore occupational musculoskeletal problems and potential risk factors among typists in a government department of Hong Kong. 170 typists were interviewed and more than 50% of the typists reported of fatigue that affected their neck and shoulder regions. Most symptoms occurred after continuous typing. Univariate analyses showed that these symptoms may be due to a poor matching between desk height and chair height. Bovenzi *et al.* (1991) studied 65 forestry operators who were repeatedly exposed to the mechanical vibration of chain-saws. A job analysis indicated that the prevalence rates of TNS and cervical syndromes were significantly higher in forestry workers than workers in health control. These results suggested that vibration stress may play an important role in contributing to the development of musculoskeletal disorders in workers who were using hand-held vibrating tools.

PREVENTIVE MEASURES

Preventive measures for OCD can be taken at both organisational and personal levels. At the organisational level, employers can conduct a series of programmes in risk identification, risk measurement, risk control and monitoring of the employees' working environments. The aims are to provide a safe and healthy working environment and to minimise the likelihood of employees developing occupational diseases and injuries at work. Occupational health and safety training programmes may be useful to achieve this aim. Preventive measures can also be taken at the personal level. Employees are required to increase their daily awareness to follow safety procedures and guidelines. Occupational health education and training are essential, e.g. changing one's posture from time to time during work in order to avoid overstraining the muscles. It is important to note that these two operational levels of preventive measures are inter-related and are equally important to maintain the good health and fitness of employees at work. Product quality and production efficiency would improve in return. In the following subsections, a number of preventive measures are explained and they are organised in a manner such that beginner will find it easy to follow.

Risk assessment / Job analysis

Risk assessment should be performed if a particular job is suspected as causing OCS. The objectives are to identify the presence of any specific risk factors in either job designs, worker behaviours or working policies (Figure 2). For example, cervicalgia is a common complaint in office workers and receptionists. In job assessment, cradling of the telephone handset is found to be a common practice in workers who are required to answer frequent telephone calls. Frequent telephone handset cradling was therefore identified to be a risk factor in cervicalgia. Beginners may find an ergonomic checklist useful for making the assessment (Pantry, 1995).

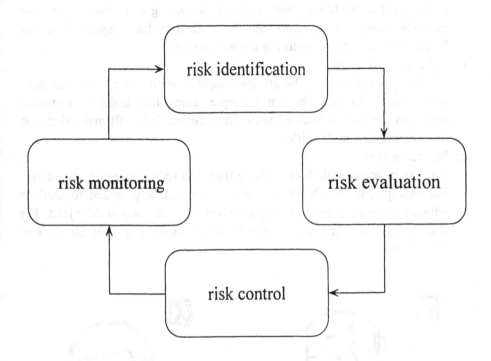

Figure 2. Cycle of occupational risk prevention.

Ergonomic principles

Ergonomics is the science of configuring working environments to suit the individual. It aims at promoting the well-being, safety and efficiency of workers by investigating human capabilities and limitations in relation to the work system, machinery or task and the physical, psychological and social environments in the workplace, and by addressing the interaction between a worker, the workplace and equipment used to perform a specific job (Isernhagen, 1995; ILO, 1982). Work design is an important area of ergonomics. Design of tools, machines, workplaces and work methods are carefully investigated in order to obtain the most appropriate solution for a particular work situation. Several principles can be used to reduce repetitive elements in the work cycle, as discussed below.

(a) Minimising repetitive motion

Work tasks will be analysed and broken down into different working components. The sequence of these components will be rearranged to spread out repetitive elements evenly in the whole working procedure or to distribute the workload over different muscle groups and joints. For example, computer operators can be advised to have regular 5-minute breaks at hourly intervals during the working day.

(b) Enlarging job scope

Similar types of jobs can be grouped together so that employees can have some variety in the job. For example, computing tasks of computer operators can be interspersed with filing duties. This will make their job less monotonous and healthy.

(c) Mechanisation

The use of appropriate tools will be useful to reduce stressful repetitions. For example, a headphone type of receiver can be provided to workers who are required to cradle a telephone handset frequently in their jobs. The risk of causing neck and shoulder muscle strain can then be reduced (Figure 3).

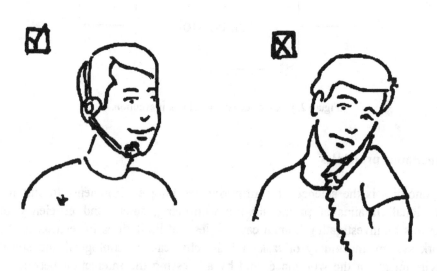

Figure 3. Correction and incorrect neck postures in telephone operator.

d) Automation

Automation is a practical and advantageous remedy for some highly repetitive operations. For example, machines can be used to perform assembly work in a production line. Workers can be re-deployed to concentrate on other duties, such as quality control, that require human judgements and discretion.

e) Postural changes

Neck and shoulder disorders have been assessed in manufacturing, construction and agricultural workers. They usually have to perform overhead work with raised arms and head titled backwards. Electromyographic (EMG) studies have demonstrated that this posture will cause a heavy load to shoulder muscles. However, the postural problems may be solved by modifying the operation of work and altering the tools or controls.

f) Job rotation

The cost of job rotation is little but it can be very effective to minimise repetitive work, particularly whenever work re-design is not possible. Job rotation provides a variety of work demands. As a result, work tasks or posture can be changed from time to time. The problem of the strain on specific musculoskeletal tissue in performing repetitive work can thus be solved. However, attention should be paid to the following factors before enforcing job rotation:

1. Sufficient time will be needed to allow workers to get used to new job in every rotation sequence,
2. Re-adjustment of skills is required as workers alternate between tasks,
3. The optimal combinations in planning job rotation, such as levels of force, frequency and grip, have not yet established.

Preventive stretching

Preventive stretching is a personal preventive measure against OCD which requires the initiation of the employees. Some simple but frequent stretching exercises can be done during work. Evidence has shown that these exercises can be very effective in reducing OCS problems in many settings. However, it is important to remember that all preventive stretching exercises should be safe and effective. Exercises should be carefully designed. Qualified experts are required to train workers to ensure they can do the exercise properly (Richardson & Eastlake, 1994). For example, an industrial physiotherapist may help to introduce appropriate neck stretching exercises to workers.

Occupational health and safety programmes and training

Effective training and proper instructions are essential to ensure employees perform their jobs safely without affecting working quality and production standards. The number and types of potentially harmful body movements should be minimised as far as possible. Risk factors contributing to OCD should be avoided. A "Worksmart" training programme should be implemented for employees so that they know how to minimise fatigue. Employees should be educated to treat themselves as "professional industrial athletes" who need to use proper work techniques and take proper care of their bodies to avoid muscle ache and pain after work. The emphasis of the programme is self-protection and how to avoid fatigue and discomfort due to work. Employers and management personnel should be aware of the work health, safety and ergonomics of their employees since high productivity and efficiency can only be achieved with a team of fit and healthy workers. Most importantly, safely working conditions will minimise occupational injuries. Enormous amounts of work compensation claims can then be avoided. (Pantry, 1995; Akass, 1994).

CONCLUSION

Most of the discussions and examples of this chapter are based on studies from the US and Sweden, where technologies and research on occupational safety and health are well developed. It is important to learn from these overseas experience in order to develop and adapt an occupational health and safety programme for our local society. In Hong Kong, the incident rate of job-related musculoskeletal diseases is increasing rapidly, especially when Hong Kong industries are getting more diversified and complicated in recent years. Therefore, occupational disorders should not be overlooked. As compared with classic treatment principles of occupational diseases, preventive medicine is found to be important because it can modify the risk factors of occupational diseases, which is more effective than treating patients' symptoms. Therefore, physiotherapists are not only required to be equipped with good therapeutic skills but are also required to ascertain job-related factors which will be helpful in preventing recurrence of symptoms. Workers can then actively participate in their jobs.

References:

Akass R. Essential health and safety for managers ~ A guide to good practice
      in the European Union. England, Gower 1994.
Bergqvist U., Wolgast E., Nilsson B., Voss M. Musculoskeletal disorders
      among visual display terminal workers: Individual, ergonomic, and
      work organizational factors. Ergonomics 1995;38:763-6.
Blader S. Neck and shoulder complaints among sewing-machine operators.
      Appl Ergon 1991;22:251-7.

Bovenzi M., Zadini A., Franzinelle A., Borgogni F. Occupational musculoskeletal disorders in the neck and upper limbs of forestry workers exposed to hand-arm vibration. Ergonomics 1991;34:547-62.

Bureau of Labour Statistics, US Department of Labour. Occupational injuries and illnesses in the United States by Industry 1993. Washington DC, US Government Printing Office 1995.

Dimberg L., Olafsson A., Stefansson E., Aagaard H., Oden A., Andersson G.B.J. The correlation between work environment and the occurrence of cervicobrachial symptoms. J Occup Med 1989;31:447-53.

Holmstrom E.B., Lindell J., Moritz U. Low back and neck/shoulder pain in construction workers: occupational work-load and psychosocial risk factors. Spine 1992;17:663-77.

HSE. Work related upper limb disorders. Sheffield, UK Health and Safety Executive (1990).

ILO. Safety-health and working conditions. Geneva, Switzerland, International Labour Office 1982.

Isernhagen S.J. The comprehensive guide to work injury management. US, An Aspen Publication 1995.

Johnsson J.A., Rubenowitz S. Risk indicators in the psychosocial and physical work environment for work-related neck, shoulder and low back symptoms: a study among blue and white collar workers in eight companies. Scan J Rehabil Med 1994;26:131-42.

Kamwendo K., Linton S.J., Moritz U. Neck and shoulder disorders in medical secretaries. Part I. Pain prevalence and risk factors. Scan J Rehabil Med 1991;23:127-33.

Linton S.J., Kamwendo K. Risk factors in the psychosocial work environment for neck and shoulder pain in secretaries. J Occup Med 1998;31:609-13.

Maeda K., Horiguchi S., Hosokawa M. History of the studies on occupational cervicobrachial disorders in Japan and remaining problems. J Hum Ergol 1982;11:17-29.

McPhee B. Musculoskeletal complaints engaged in repetitive work in fixed postures. Edinburgh, UK, International perspectives in physical therapy-ergonomics 1990.

National Occupational Health and Safety Commission. Guidance note for the prevention of occupational overuse syndrome in keyboard employment. Canberra, AGPS 1989.

Okawara S., Nibbelink D. Vertebral artery occlusion following hyperextension and rotation of the head. Stroke 1974;5:640-2.

Pantry S. Occupational Health. London, Chapman & Hall 1995.

Putz-Anderson V. Cumulative trauma disorders: a manual for musculoskeletal diseases of the upper limb. Bristol, PA, Taylor and Francis 1992.

Ranney. Chronic musculoskeletal injuries in the workplace. Philadelphia, WB Saunders Company 1997.

Richardson B., Eastlake A. Physiotherapy in occupational health. UK, Butterworth Heinemann 1994.

Sakakibara H., Miyao M., Kondo T., Yamada S. Overhead work and shoulder-neck pain in orchard farmers harvesting pears and apples. Ergonomics 1995;38:700-6.

Salvendy G., Smith M.J. Machine pain and occupational stress. New York, Taylor and Francis 1981.

Viikara-Juntura E., Riihimaki H., Toll S., Videman T., Mutanen P. Neck trouble in machine operating, dynamic physical work and sedentary work: a prospective study on occupational and individual risk factors. J Clin Epidemiol 1994;47:1411-22.

Yu I.T.S., Wong T.W. Musculoskeletal problems among VDU workers in a Hong Kong bank. Occup Med 1996;46:275-80.

Yu I.T.S., Tsang Y.Y., Liu T.Y. Self reported musculoskeletal problems amongst typist and possible risks factors. J Human Ergol 1993;22:83-93.

Suggested reading list:

Schuldt K., Ekholm J., Harms-Ringdahl K., Nemeth G., Arborelius U.P. Effects of changes in sitting work posture on neck and shoulder muscle activity. Ergonomics 1986;29:1525-37.

Snjiders C.J., Hoek van Dijke G.A., Roosch E.R. A biomechanical model for the analysis of the cervical spine in static posture. J Biomech 1991;24:783-92.

CHAPTER 10

ERGONOMICS OF THE SHOULDER AND NECK

Simon S. Yeung

INTRODUCTION

Work-related musculoskeletal disorder (WMSD) is one of the most common musculoskeletal disorders that therapists will encounter in orthopaedic practice. This chapter focuses on the effects of WMSDs on the work force, the epidemiology of shoulder and neck disorders, possible causative models in the development of the disorders and the ergonomic principles in the prevention and control of these disorders.

OCCUPATIONAL INJURIES AND WORK-RELATED MUSCULO-SKELETAL DISORDERS

The cost and prevalence of occupational injuries and disease are enormous in all industrialised countries. A population survey undertaken by the Australian Bureau of Statistics revealed that between 160,000 and 220,000 workers have been absent from work for at least one day in any given two week period and the estimate cost of work-related injuries and diseases in 1992-1993 was $20 billion!

The five most prevalent work-related injuries and diseases leading to five or more days off work are sprains and strains, open wounds, fractures, contusion and crushing and disorders of the muscles and tendons (Industry Commission, 1995). Kuorinka and Forcier (1995) defined WMSDs as musculoskeletal disorders and diseases which have proven or hypothetical work-related components. The National Institute of Occupational Safety and Health (NIOSH) had classified musculoskeletal disorders as one of the top ten occupational disorders in the United States (NIOSH 1987).

Among all the WMSDs, injuries at the upper limbs are by far the most common. These kinds of injuries had been defined as Occupational Overuse

Syndrome (OOS), also known as Repetitive Strain Injury (RSI) in Australia, Cumulative Trauma Disorders (CTD) in North America and Occupational Cervico-brachial Disorder (OCD) in Japan. It is, in general, a collective term to describe a range of conditions which are characterised by discomfort or pain in the muscles, tendons and other soft tissues at the upper extremities, with or without definite physical signs.

This can be broadly divided into two main categories in which the first group consists of localised, definable conditions that are well understood. Typical examples are carpal tunnel syndrome, DeQuervain's syndrome, tenosynovitis and shoulder tendinitis. The second group is less localised and the pathology is less understood. A typical example is tension neck syndrome. Table 1 summarises a number of different disorders commonly occurring in the shoulder and neck region.

Table 1. Examples of work-related shoulder-neck disorders.

Muscle problems	Neck myalgia
	Trapezius myalgia
	Tension neck syndrome
Tendon problems	Rotator cuff tendinitis
	Bicipital tendinitis
Nerve problems	Thoracic outlet syndrome
	Cervical spondylosis

Epidemiology of work-related shoulder and neck disorders

In the identification of occupational disease, there usually exists a cause-effect relationship between the hazards and the diseases (e.g. asbestos and asbestosis). This cause-effect relationship is usually less obvious in work-related diseases or disorders. The causes are multifactorial with work environment and the nature of work being the main contributing factors. Risk factors are usually defined as job attributes that increase the probability of WMSDs.

CTD in the shoulder and neck region are typical work-related diseases of which the cause-effect relationship cannot be easily established. The term "cumulative" indicates that the disorders usually develop gradually over a period of time as a result of repeated stress. "Trauma" implies injury resulting from mechanical stress and "disorders" refers to physical ailments rather than a specific medical entity (Putz-Anderson, 1993).

In the review of epidemiological studies related to CTD, problems are usually non-specific and have been defined either by subjective symptomatic reports or confirmation with medical findings. As such, the prevalence rate is generally lower when using physical examination rather than based on the workers' subjective report. For instance, Hagberg and Wegman (1987) reported that the prevalence rate of medical diagnosed tension neck syndrome among male industrial workers in United States was 1.9%. However, CTD cases from symptoms as been reported to have a prevalence rate of up to 50% (Hales *et al.*, 1994). Putz-Anderson (1993) identified four categories of work-related risk factors which might cause CTD. They are exertion level, repetition, posture and lack of rest. In addition to the work-related risk factors, personal factors such as age, gender, past history of acute trauma (Bergqvist *et al.*, 1995) and sports and hobbies (Lehman, 1988) have also been shown to influence the occurrence of work-related shoulder and neck disorder.

Dose-response model of WMSDs

Armstrong and his co-workers (1993) proposed a dose-response model to relate various risk factors that contributed to the pathogenesis of work-related musculoskeletal disorders. This dose-response model is based on four sets of cascading and interacting variables, namely exposure, dose, capacity and response. The effects of the variables at one level would produce a cascading effect at the next level. In this model, "exposure" refers to the external work environment which produces internal "doses" in the worker.

Workplace organisation, environment and job demand are typical examples of "exposure". "Dose" is the consequence of the external factors that lead to internal changes of the body. These could be mechanical stress and deformations of soft tissues due to overexertion and the repetitive nature of the work, physiological energy expenditure, as well as psychological stress induced by the job. The "response" corresponds to the effect of the dose caused by exposure. Depending on the nature and the intensity of the dose, the response could either resulting in an increase or decrease of an individual's dose tolerance (capacity). "Capacity" is thus the worker's physical and psychological ability to resist destabilisation of the system resulted from the doses. This dose-response model highlighted the multifactorial nature of work-related musculoskeletal disorders and its complexity in nature. The interaction between exposure, dose, response and capacity are cascading and accumulating in nature.

Shoulder and neck muscle related disorders

Muscle soreness, ache and pain are the most common complaints of work-related shoulder and neck problems. Muscle soreness is an early sign of local muscle fatigue. If the problem cannot be properly addressed, it may progress to muscle ache and pain. A sustained static loading, as low as 5% of the maximum voluntary contraction for one hour (Sjøgaard *et al.*, 1986; Sjøgaard *et al.*, 1988), has been shown to induce muscle fatigue. Hagberg (1984) postulated that the causes of shoulder and neck muscle related disorders could be due to (1) heavy physical exertion or eccentric contraction of the trapezius muscle which lead to rupture of the muscle's Z band; (2) decrease in local blood flow due to frequent dynamic low level of contraction (10~20% MVC) and (3) disturbance of energy metabolism due to long term static contraction.

WORK-RELATED RISK FACTORS

Tremendous efforts have been made by health and safety and ergonomic professionals to establish the risk factors associated with the development of shoulder and neck disorders. Most of the epidemiological studies showed that frequent or prolonged repetitive movements, forceful exertions, awkward postures, static muscle loading, cold temperatures and vibration are the main risk factors associated with the prevalence of such problems. A recent critical review (Bernard *et al.*, 1997) showed strong evidence of the causal relationship between highly repetitive work, forceful exertion and high levels of static contraction, prolonged static loads and/or awkward working postures, and the occurrence of shoulder and neck disorders. The effects of these risk factors are discussed below.

Repetition

Ohlsson *et al.*, (1995) conducted a cross-sectional study of female industrial assembly-line workers whose work routines involve highly repetitive tasks, with a work cycle of less than 30 seconds. The tasks required a work posture of intermittent neck flexion, and with the shoulder in an elevated and abducted position. This group of workers was compared with a group of former assembly workers and another group of workers whose jobs do not require repetitive neck and shoulder movement. The results revealed an odd ratio of 4.6 for the association between repetition and work-related shoulder and neck disorders. In a three-year study, the postures and complaints of female electronic workers with highly repetitive and combined with awkward neck and shoulder postures were assessed. In a two-year follow-up, the rate of repetition of neck flexion per hour was found to be a strong predictor for the deterioration of the neck disorders. The mean number of neck forward flexion per hour was 728 and the work cycle time varied between 4.7 and 9.1 min (Kilbom *et al.*, 1986; Kilbom and Persson 1987, Jonsson *et al.*, 1988). Occupations that required workers to perform repetitive shoulder and neck movement include Visual Display Terminal (VDT) workers, dentists, electronic assembly workers and sewing machine operators (Bernard *et al.*, 1997).

Exertion level

Work activities that involve strenuous work in the upper arms and neck will cause pressure on the trapezius and neck musculature. The amount of weight has been found to be a contributing factor to shoulder disorders. Wells *et al.*, (1983) showed a 4-kg increase in bag weight of the letter carriers increased the prevalence rate of shoulder and neck pain from 13% to 23%. This study also compared letter carriers with gas meter readers and postal clerks whose jobs do not require heavy loads on the shoulder musculature. Their results showed a significant difference in the reported rate of neck pain between letter carriers and the other two job categories. Quantification of muscle load is usually done through an electromyographic (EMG) measurement or as a percentage of MVC. It has been shown that symptomatic subjects showed higher EMG activities in the trapezius than the pain free subjects (Erdelyi *et al.*, 1988).

Work posture

Kilbom and Persson (1987) showed that a shoulder abduction of more than 30° contributed to work related shoulder disorders. Ohlsson *et al.*, (1995) showed a significant association between neck and neck/shoulder disorders with neck flexion of more than 15° and arm abduction of more than 60°. Power spectral analysis of the shoulder flexors and abductors revealed that fatigue onset on the shoulder flexors depends on the angle of shoulder flexion. When the vertical height placement of the hand were 5 cm, 30 cm and 57 cm above the table top, the onset time of fatigue had been reported to be 20 mins, 9 mins and 5 mins (Chaffin, 1973) respectively. For the shoulder abductors, fatigue occurred at 68 mins, 25 mins, 10 mins and 7 mins when the shoulder was at 30°, 60°, 90° and 120° of shoulder abduction (Chaffin, 1973). Sustained activities in the same position had also been shown to be correlated with the occurrence of tendon related disorder in the shoulder region, e.g. supraspinatus tendinitis (Herberts *et al.*, 1984). Occupations that involve frequent, extreme and awkward shoulder and neck posture include fish workers, fruit pickers, assembly line workers and garment workers (Bernard *et al.*, 1997).

While efforts had been made to relate the occurrence and prevalence of work-related musculoskeletal disorders of the shoulder and neck, it has to be noted that risk factors are interacting with each other as discussed in Armstrong *et al.*'s (1993) dose-dependent model. As such, modelling has been used to relate work-related risk factors to the occurrence of the musculoskeletal disorders. For instance, based on available evidence, high repetition, excessive forces and awkward postures have a strong association with the development of work-related disorders of the upper limbs. Genaidy *et al* (1993) developed a stress index which is an interaction between the effects of repetition, force and posture. The stress index provided recommendations of maximum permissible limits which are essentially based on the approach of the NIOSH (1981) manual material handling assessment.

ERGONOMIC PRINCIPLES IN THE PREVENTION OF WORK-RELATED SHOULDER AND NECK DISORDERS

The word "Ergonomics" originates from the Greek *ergo* (work) and *nomos* (rules, law). It bears the meaning of law governing work. Ergonomics is a scientific discipline to study the interaction between the human at work and the working environment. The main objectives are to enhance the effectiveness and efficiency of work and activities and to improve work safety, reduce fatigue and stress, increase comfort, job satisfaction and better quality of life. The approach of ergonomics is a systematic application of relevant information about human physical characteristics, behaviour and motivation to the design of products, work procedures and environments in which people work. With the enactment of the Occupational Safety and Health (OSH) Ordinance on 23rd May 1997 (Hong Kong Government Gazette, 1997), there is a major breakthrough in the work health and safety policy in Hong Kong. This represents a shift of emphasis from only safety to both safety and health of workers at work. As such, physiotherapists should be equipped with a basic knowledge of ergonomic principles so as to expand the services to this group of clientele.

Ergonomic principles

The basic principles in the management of work-related musculoskeletal disorders include (1) risk factor identification and assessment; (2) work site analysis followed by risk control measures; (3) rehabilitation and (4) training and education.

Work-related risk factors that are associated with the development of shoulder-neck disorders have been discussed in the previous sections. These factors when considered in the work scenario should include (1) the types of work (nature of jobs) in which workers are involved; (2) working posture; (3) the use of repeated movements and forces; (4) the workstation design; (5) work organisation and (6) the physical profile of the workers.

Ergonomic work site analysis

Worksite analysis is a systematic safety and health review. It assists in the identification of workers' jobs and workstations that may contribute to the risk factors. It should begin with reviewing company records to identify patterns of injuries and identification of potential jobs and workstations that may cause musculoskeletal hazards. The analysis should then be related to relevant research survey statistics. The company records that would help to identify the risk factors include (1) accident reports or incident reports; (2) safety committee reports; (3) job descriptions; (3) employee complaints and employee turnover rate. These factors can also be ascertained from a survey on workers work health and musculoskeletal discomfort. The work site assessment should address the causes of particular risk factors. The areas of assessment should include work posture, equipment and tools, workstation layout, work organisation and physical work environment.

Work posture

A good working posture for the shoulders should allow the shoulders to be relaxed in a neutral position and the upper arms to be close to the sides of the body. Pressure on the shoulder will increase with sustained shoulder and/or arm elevation. Measures that can be taken include supporting the weight of the object/tool being held and decreasing the speed or the frequency of the task required and the repetition of the task.

Equipment and tools design

The equipment and tools should be designed to fit the individual user and fulfil the specific demands of the work task. Good tool design would allow workers to perform their work with limbs in neutral positions. The tools selected should be of the optimal weight to perform the task. A heavy tool will increase static loading on the shoulder muscle. The handgrip of the tool should not add pressure to tissues and joints.

Workstation layout

Work requirements stipulate the height of the work surface. In essence, the work surface should be either below the elbow if the task requires considerable muscle strength or slightly above the elbow for ordinary deskwork. For work requiring manual precision, the forearms should be well supported and above the elbow level. The visual requirements of tasks determine the head and neck posture of the worker. Therefore, due consideration should be given to visual acuity of the workers, the accuracy of the task required and the lighting condition. The workstation layout should also conform to the anthropometric data of the working groups.

Work organisation

Good work organisation will minimise both the physical and psychological stress on workers. Task rotation, enrichment and automation should be considered to reduce the effects of monotonous, sustained and repetitive activities. A good balance between work and rest helps to prevent overexertion and development of muscle fatigue. A work adjustment period may be beneficial for newly employed staff.

Physical work environment

A good physical work environment will not only increase the efficiency of workers, but can also minimise fatigue and musculoskeletal injuries caused by adverse physical conditions. The physical work environment assessment should thus be an integral part of work site analysis. This should include noise level, atmospheric and lighting conditions. Parsons (1995) presented a summary of the international ergonomics standards of speech communication, danger signals, lighting, vibration and surface temperatures and is a good reference on this issue.

Risk control

Risk control is a process to eliminate or minimise risk through implementation of appropriate measures. In shoulder and neck disorders, this is similar to the hazard management approach in which the hierarchy of risk control should be the elimination of the hazard, substitution of the hazard, engineering control (e.g. provision of balances for heavy power tools), administrative control (e.g. job rotation, training) and provision of personal protective equipment (e.g. anti-vibration gloves).

Work rehabilitation

The causes of work-related shoulder and neck disorders involve many aspects of the work environment and the nature of work. Early reporting of symptoms will aid the identification of risky tasks that may affect workers at work. Medical treatment and rehabilitation should commence as early as possible. The aim of work rehabilitation is to assist workers in regaining their functional, physical and psychological capacities. A work hardening programme is commonly used to improve these capacities. This is a well-structured, goal-oriented programme that utilises real or simulated work activities and are graded progressively to improve an individual's biomechanical, neuromuscular, cardiovascular and psychosocial functions. In the rehabilitation process, therapists should always consider the possibilities of early return to work, and a functional capacity evaluation can assist in deciding whether the worker should return to work with either alternate work placement, modified duties, work trail or full duties.

Training and education

Training and education is an integral part of the whole preventive strategy. Workers should be provided with information on the causes and possible risk factors of shoulder-neck disorders and the early signs and symptoms of such disorders. They should be trained and educated on the correct use of tools and equipment, good work posture and body mechanics, as well as the importance of breaks from work and tasks rotation.

CONCLUSION

The causes of work-related shoulder-neck disorders are multifactorial with work environment and the nature of work being the main contributing factors. Work-related risk factors that show strong association with the development of work-related shoulder-neck disorders are high repetition of work activities, excessive force and awkward postures. Ergonomics aims to identify these risk factors at work and implement appropriate measures to minimise the risks. A good understanding of ergonomic principles and their systematic application are therefore essential in the prevention and management of work-related shoulder-neck disorders.

References:

Armstrong T.J., Buckle P., Fine L.J., Jonsson B., Kilbom A., Kuorinka I.A., Silverstein A., Sjøgaard G., Viikari-Juntura E.R. A conceptual model for work-related neck and upper-limb musculoskeletal disorders. Scand J Work Environ Health 1993;19:73-84.

Bergqvist U., Wolgast E., Nilsson B. Musculoskeletal disorders among visual display terminal workers: individual, ergonomics and work organisation factors. Ergonomics. 1995;38:763-76.

Bernard B.P., Putz-Anderson V., Burt S.E. *et al.* Musculoskeletal disorders (MSDs) and workplace factors: A critical review of epidemiological evidence for work-related musculoskeletal disorders of the neck, upper extremity, and low back. U.S. Department of Health and Human Services, Public Health Service, Centers for Disease Control and Prevention, National Institute for Occupational Safety and Health, Cincinnati,OH (http://www.cdc.gov/ niosh/ergosci1.htm)1997.

Chaffin D. Localized muscle fatigue: definition and measurement. J Occup Med 1973;15:346-54.

Erdelyi A., Sihvonen T., Helin P., Hänninen O. Shoulder strain in keyboard workers and its alleviation by arm supports. Int Arch Occup Environ Health 1988;60:119-24.

Genaidy A., Al-Shedi A., Shell R. Ergonomic risk assessment: Preliminary guidelines for analysis of repetition, force and posture. J Human Ergol 1993;22:45-55.

Hagberg M., Wegman D. Prevalence rates and odds ratios of shoulder-neck diseases in different occupational groups. Br J Ind Med 1987;44:602-10.

Hagberg M. Occupational musculoskeletal stress and disorders of the neck and shoulder: a review of possible pathophysiology. Int Arch Occup Environ Health. 1984;53:269-78.

Hales T., Sauter S., Peterson M.., Fine L., Putz-Anderson V., Schleifer L., Ochs T., Bernard B. Musculoskeletal disorders among visual display terminal users in a telecommunications company. Ergonomics. 1994;37:1603-21.

Herberts P., Kadefors R., Högfors C., Sigholm G. Shoulder pain in industry: an epidemiological study on welders. Clin Orthop 1984;191:166-78.

Hong Kong Government Gazette. Occupational Safety and Health Ordinance. 1997.

Industry Commission. Work, Health and Safety, Inquiry into occupational health and safety, Report No. 47, Vol. 1, AGPS, Canberra, Australia. 1995.

Jonsson B., Persson J., Kilbom A. Disorders of the cervicobrachial region among female workers in the electronics industry: A two year follow-up. Int J Ind Ergon 1988;3:1-12.

Kilbom A., Persson J., Jonsson B. Disorders of the cervicobrachial region among female workers in the electronics industry. Int J Ind Ergon 1986;1:37-47.

Kilbom Å., Persson J. Work technique and its consequences for musculoskeletal disorders. Ergonomics. 1987;30:273-9.

Kuorinka I., Forcier L. Work Related Musculoskeletal Disorders (WMSDs): A reference Book for Prevention. London: Taylor and Francis, 1995.

Lehman R.C. Shoulder pain in the competitive tennis player. Clin Sports Med 1988;7:309-27.

National Institute for Occupational Safety and Health. Work practices guide for manual lifting, NIOSH Technical Report DHHS (NIOSH) Publication No. 81-122, 1981.

National Institute of Occupational Safety and Health. Surveillance of Occupational Illness and Injury in the United States: Current Perspectives and Future Directions. U.S. Dept. of Health and Human Services. 1987.

Ohlsson K., Attewell R., Paisson B. Repetitive industrial work and neck and upper limb disorders in females. Am J Ind Med 1995;27:731-47.

Parsons K. Ergonomics of the physical environment: International ergonomics standards concerning speech communication, danger signals, lighting, vibration and surface temperatures. Appl Ergono 1995;26:281-92.

Putz-Anderson V. Cumulative Trauma Disorders. A manual for Musculoskeletal Diseases for the Upper Limbs. London, Taylor and Francis 1993.

Sjogaard G., Kiens B., Jorgensen K., Saltin B. Intramuscular pressure, EMG and blood flow during low-level prolonged static contraction in man. Acta Physiol Scand 1986;128:475-84.

Sjøgaard G., Savard G., Juel C. Muscle blood flow during isometric activity and its relation to muscle fatigue. Eur J Appl Physiol Occup Physiol 1988;57:327-35.

Wells J., Zipp J., Schuette P., McEleney J. Musculoskeetal disorders among letter carriers. J Occup Med 1983;25:81.

CHAPTER 11

SPORT INJURIES OF THE CERVICAL SPINE

Candy Wu

INTRODUCTION

Cervical spine injuries in sports can be classified into either catastrophic or non-catastrophic injury. Catastrophic sport injury is defined as any injury leading to either a permanent or transient functional and neurological deficit (Harries *et al.*, 1994). In addition, there are also life-threatening cases, when severe fractures and/or dislocations compromise the spinal cord. Fortunately, the percentage of catastrophic and fatal cervical injuries is not high. To date, there appears to be no statistics available which address the number of catastrophic and non-catastrophic cervical sport injuries in Hong Kong. According to record of the Sport Medicine Department at the Hong Kong Sports Institute in 1997, 0.9% of the athletes who were treated by the sport physiotherapists of the Institute suffered from neck problems. They were either gymnasts, windsurfers, rowers or badminton players. Gymnasts ranked at the top of the list (25%), followed by windsurfers (16.7%) and finally rowers and badminton players (both 10.5%). The problems they encountered included acute wry neck, sprains, strains and chronic wear and tear. However, as some high risk sports such as diving, equestrian, rugby, American football, ice hockey and skydiving, are not popular in Hong Kong, the number of catastrophic cervical spine injuries is expected to be low.

MECHANISM OF INJURY

There is some controversy regarding which mechanisms contribute most to the catastrophic cervical sport injuries. Some suggest that hyperflexion and hyperextension are the predominant forces causing the injuries, while others believe that axial loading or vertex impact is the most frequent cause of serious cervical injuries (Harries *et al.*, 1994; Tator *et al.*, 1984; Torg *et al.*, 1979;

1991a; 1991b; 1993). Despite this controversy, it is generally agreed that minor sprains and strains of the cervical spine are the most common sport injuries in the neck. For both catastrophic and non-catastrophic injuries, the usual mechanisms are the following.

- Sudden hyperflexion may cause a compression fracture at the anterior cervical vertebrae and ligament injuries at the posterior side of the cervical spine. Sometimes, fractures of joint processes and joint capsule injuries may occur. Many authors have suggested that hyperflexion can cause catastrophic cervical spine injuries in some sports, such as rugby, diving, wrestling and American football. However, some researchers argued that injury of the cervical spine through hyperflexion alone is anatomically impossible (Peterson *et al.*, 1992).

- Hyperextension injuries may occur in contact sports, falls and deceleration of dynamic flexion movements. Damage of anterior discs and ligaments and compressive fracture of the posterior vertebral bodies may result from hyperextension injuries (Peterson *et al.*, 1992). Some authors have suggested that hyperflexion and hyperextension are the two dominant forces producing most types of cervical lesions with cord damage in American football, rugby, diving and general sports. However, according to Torg *et al.* (1991b), only a small percentage of injuries leading to quadriplegia or fracture/dislocation without quadriplegia, were contributed by hyperextension.

- Axial compression is the most popular mechanism discussed and investigated, especially in American footballers, swimmers and divers (Harries *et al.*, 1994; Torg *et al.*, 1979; 1991a; 1991b; 1993). Injuries can result from falls, violent collision with an opponent or with surrounding objects, when the head hits the pool floor in diving, or crashing into the boards head first in ice hockey. In such situations, the fragile cervical spine is compressed between the decelerated head and the continued momentum of the body. Injuries have been reported even at velocities as low as 3.1 m/s with only a fraction of the torso mass loading upon the cervical spine (Torg *et al.*, 1991b). According to Torg *et al.* (1991a; 1991b; 1993), axial loading of the cervical spine commonly occurs when the neck is slightly flexed (approximately 30°).

  The significance of this point is that the normal cervical lordosis is straightened and the spine is converted into a segmented column. With the impact travelling along the longitudinal axis of a straight spine, energy is initially absorbed by intervertebral discs and neck muscles. When a maximum compressive deformation is reached, angular deformation and buckling will then occur. Subluxation, facet dislocation or fracture dislocation may result from the failure of discs, ligaments and bones. Bauze and Ardan (1978) demonstrated that failure in facet joint and posterior ligament occurred when axial loads were applied to cadaveric spines. When the lower portion of the spine was flexed and fixed and the upper cervical spine was extended with freedom to move forward, vertical compression may produce bilateral dislocation of the facet joints without fracture. If lateral tilt or axial rotation occurs, a unilateral dislocation may produce. All forces observed in these injuries are less than those required for bony failure and allow facet dislocation without associated bony pathology (Torg *et al.*, 1993). In an experiment done by Bauze (1978), the maximum vertical loading required for forward dislocation was 1,420N. Other literature review reported that the limits of axial compressive loading in human cervical vertebral bodies were between 3,340 to 4,450N. The cervical spine is able to sustain heavy load under direct compression when it is straight (i.e. loss of normal lordosis). If the spine is not straight, axial load will result in asymmetric loading and cause bending movements and deformation (Torg *et al.*, 1991b). In Burstein *et al.*'s (1982) impact study with an anatomic model, they found that helmets was not a reliable means to absorb the kinetic energy of the torso. The trunk continued to exert this energy on the neck until a sufficient amount of energy was stored to damage the cervical spine. They concluded that the best way to prevent this kind of injury is to avoid axial loading. Proper techniques of tackling and diving should be stressed and they should not be forsaken just because helmets have been used. Helmets can only protect the skull to a certain extent, not the neck (Torg *et al.*, 1991b).

Fortunately, most head impacts do not cause cervical spine injuries. Analysis of the biomechanical and clinical literature shows that the flexibility of the cervical spine frequently allows the head and neck to flex or extend out of the path of the torso and then escape from severe injury. Restriction of neck movements will therefore increase the risk of cervical injury. Proper sporting techniques, flexibility training and strengthening exercises should be emphasised to be a major part of the injury prevention programme (Torg *et al.*, 1991b).

- High velocity accidents can occur during car racing, skiing, speed skating and snowboarding. Collision will cause serious cervical injury and sometimes even death. Whiplash type injuries can also occur when the neck is suddenly and violently extended and then flexed. Ligaments, bones, muscle injuries and fracture/dislocation may also occur.

- Forced excessive range of motion, such as lateral flexion and rotation, can also cause cervical spine injuries. This mechanism may occur during wrestling or judo, when an athlete is forced into a awkward position by an opponent. This movement may also occur in badminton, when a player tries to hit a shuttlecock such that there is excessive neck movements, instead of moving the other parts of his/her body. Fracture/dislocation are unlikely in these situations, but muscles, ligaments and nerves may be compromised.

- Brachial plexus injury may occur when compression or traction force is exerted on the cervical spine. Injuries by compression are called "burners" and those by traction are known as "stingers". Some authors may refer to these injuries as "pinched nerve syndrome". Brachial plexus is formed from the ventral rami of C5-T1 spinal nerves. When it is injured, the classical symptoms include upper limb numbness, pins and needles, burning pain and weakness. Occasionally, the dysethesia is bilateral. The history usually involves an ipsilateral or contralateral shoulder blow that may be associated with cervical spine extension, lateral flexion or both.

BRACHIAL PLEXUS INJURIES

Brachial plexus injuries are not common in sports, except in American football in which body collision may occur. Another sport that has been reported to have a high rate of brachial plexus injury rate is mountaineering. This is because heavy backpacks are carried, which can cause compression injury (Figure 1) (Harries *et al.*, 1994; Johnson *et al.*, 1994; Reid, 1992; Torg *et al.*, 1991b). Fracture of the clavicle with exuberant callus formation can also be a source of brachial plexus compression. Moreover, hypertrophic clavicle non-union, generally in the middle of the clavicle, can produce brachial plexus compression. Early treatment of acute clavicle fractures, with the use of a figure of eight bandage, can also result in the same problem. Occasionally, a fractured clavicle fragment may encroach on the plexus causing symptoms (Torg *et al.*, 1991b). A large cervical rib may increase the risk of athletes suffering burners and stingers. Its presence will narrow the interscalene triangle and affect the angulation of the subclavian artery and the lower trunk of the brachial plexus. When the cervical rib is more than 5.5 cm in length, it may cause abnormal stretching to the 7th cervical nerve root, especially during circumduction of the arm or forced lateral flexion of the neck with depression of the shoulder (Reid, 1992).

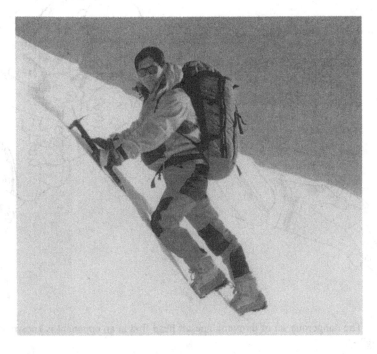

Figure 1. Heavy packs can cause brachial plexus compression injury in mountaineerers.
(photo : courtesy by Alan Chu)

AMERICAN FOOTBALL

Due to the popularity of American football, as well as its injury rate, this type
of sport has drawn a lot of researchers' attention in the USA. Figures have
shown that defensive backs and linebackers who tackle with the top of their
heads have the highest injury rate leading to permanent quadriplegia. It is
particularly true because of the dangerous act of throwing oneself head first at
an opponent. This is known as "spearing" (Figure 2), because of its similarity
to the spear (Nelson, 1993).   In 1976, the National Collegiate Athletic
Associations and the National Federation of High School Athletic Associations
adopted special rules to ban this spearing motion and the use of helmet top to
check the initial contact point during tackling or blocking. As a result, a
dramatic decrease in cervical spine injury was noted between 1976 and 1987
(Harries *et al.*, 1994; Torg *et al.*, 1979; 1991a; 1991b; 1993).

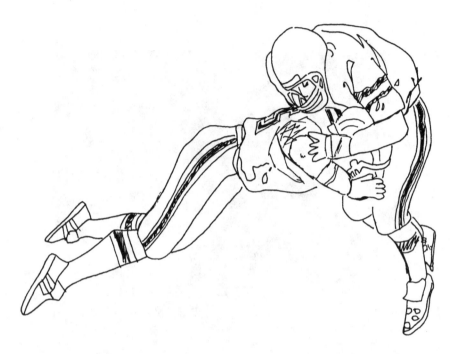

Figure 2. The dangerous act of throwing oneself head first at an opponent is known as "spearing".

RUGBY

The rate of cervical spine injury in rugby depends on its popularity in that particular country. For example, rugby has raised the concern of more researchers in the United Kingdom, New Zealand and Australia than in any other countries. When people mention rugby, they may either refer to the rugby union, rugby league or Australian rules. Although a rugby ball look the same everywhere, the rules and number of players are different in various countries. Therefore, injury patterns may differ from place to place. Taylor and Coolican (Torg, 1991b) did a comprehensive study of spinal cord injury in rugby. This study included Australian rules, rugby league, the rugby union and soccer. They found that most of the cervical spine injuries happened in scrums, particularly in rugby league. Tackling was found to be the major cause of the injury. In Australian rules, most of the players were injured in collisions whereas players generally do not hold the ball in their hands. Scrum (also known as scrummage and scrimmage) is a means of restarting play, usually following an infringement (Figure 3). At least five players must form the scrum, but usually all eight forwards players interlock in a 3-4-1 format. As two sets of the front row forwards players interlock with each other, injury can occur during ruck and maul. Ruck is a scrimmage formed by the opposing sets of forwards around the ball as it has been grounded. Maul is a scrimmage of players from both teams around a player carrying the ball. If he drops the ball to the ground, the maul then becomes a ruck.

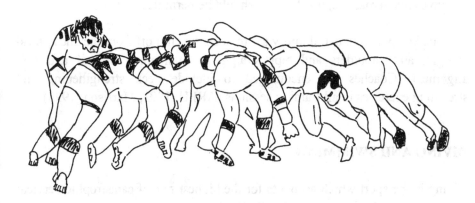

Figure 3. Scrum ~ Two sets of front row forwards interlock with each other.
(Illustration by Tony Yip)

Figures show that players may incur cervical spine injury during ruck and maul, but the number of reported injuries is less than those in scrum and tackling (Silver *et al.*, 1998; Torg, 1991b). As the number of players (15) in a rugby union is larger than that of a rugby league (13) and Australian rules do not include scrums, rucks and mauls, the number of injuries in scrums is very high (Torg, 1991b). "Depowering " of the scrum is one of the most important issues in reducing injuries. The strength of the forwards, especially the hookers (the middle forward) is critical because if there is a large discrepancy in strength between two opposing hookers, injury is likely to occur (Silver *et al.*, 1992; Torg 1991b).   Correct techniques are also essential to prevent injury. The following engagement sequence for rugby union should be strictly observed (ARFU, 1993; Marrison, 1993):

1. Crouch:
    To establish body position, the knees should be slightly bent and the upper body should incline from the hip. Shoulders should not be lower than the hips. The head should be kept straight with the chin up.

2. Touch:
    To gauge distance, touch the upper arm of the opposite prop with the outside arm.

3. Pause:
    It allows players to balance and assume a position to maximise safety.

4. Engage:
    The front rows of players will engage shoulder to shoulder after the referee
    gives his verbal cue, no charging should be permitted.

The key points to avoid injury are to keep the chin off from the chest, head
straight, and shoulders and hips straight to maintain a normal and safe
alignment. Coaches are encouraged to include neck strengthening and
stretching exercises in all training sessions (ARFU, 1993; Marrison, 1993)

DIVING AND SWIMMING

Diving is the sport which accounts for the highest rate of catastrophic cervical
spine injury (Harries *et al.*, 1994). Wedge and compression fractures are
commonly caused when people dive and hit the bottom of the pool or seabed.
Drowning may occasionally occur when the diver's spinal cord is damaged
and a quadriplegia sets in under water. In a study performed by Blanksby *et al.*
(1997), they found that the highest incidence rate of diving injuries occurred in
10~14 years old boys and in swimming pools with a pool depth less than 1.52
m. However, injuries are rare if the pool depth is between 0.46 m and 0.61 m.
These results suggest that education is very important, especially among
youngsters. One should not dive if the water depth is less than 1.52 m because
deceleration cannot occur. Pools should not be designed with a sudden change
in depth. Inexperienced divers are a high risk group because of their poor
diving techniques and judgement. Swimmers should not practise racing using
the shallow end of the pool as their starting point. Therefore, some
neurosurgeons promoted a diving technique with a motto of "feet first, first
time". They claimed that spinal cord injury had greatly decreased since this
diving technique had been used (Torg, 1991b).

GYMNASTICS

Most cervical injuries in gymnasts are found to be associated with trampoline
and minitrampoline (Chalmers *et al.*, 1994; Harries, 1994). Cases of
quadriplegia and even deaths were also reported. Chalmers *et al.*, (1994) found
that 2 deaths and 2098 hospitalisations were related to this sport in New
Zealand from 1979 to 1988. Also, the annual hospitalisation rate due to this

sport increased from 3.1 to 9.3 per 100,000 population from 1979 to 1988. Among these hospitalised patients, 71% of them were injured while using home trampolines and 80% of them fell from the trampoline to surrounding surface. Fractures were the most common type of injury (68%), yet catastrophic injuries were less frequent.

According to a literature review done by Torg (1991b), 114 catastrophic cervical injuries due to trampolines and minitrampolines were reported from 1960 to 1990. Types of injuries include vertical body compression-burst fractures, facet dislocations or subluxations and fracture/dislocations associated with intervertebral discs herniations. Some people believe that most of the injuries are caused by inexperienced athletes, careless spotters, inadequate support and poor equipment standards and maintenance. However, data shows that victims could be experienced athletes. Somersaults were found to be the most common manoeuvres leading to injuries. Therefore, some suggested that even highly trained athletes should not use the trampoline without proper supervision. Some proposed that trampolines should be completely banned in recreational, educational or competitive gymnastics (Harries *et al.*, 1994; Torg, 1991b). Therefore, the question of whether the trampoline should be banned from physical education programmes remains controversial.

EQUESTRIAN SPORTS

Horse riding is very different from the other sports mentioned previously, because good co-operation between the rider and the horse is required. The rider can be thrown off from the horse when it either fails to cross a large obstacle or responds unpredictably to the rider's order. Cervical spine injuries may then occur.

Cervical fractures are generally caused by hyperflexion of the neck. In particular, compressed fractures of the vertebral bodies with fracture or dislocation of facet joints are relatively common. These injuries are usually unstable because both the anterior and posterior elements of the vertebral body are damaged. Axial loading is, however, uncommon because riders tend to fall with their upper arms extended with their necks in flexion or extension.

Brachial plexus injuries may occur when riders fail to release the reins or saddle when they are thrown off horses. These injuries are usually stretching injuries and can be treated satisfactorily with conservative treatment (Torg, 1991b). Nelson *et al.* (1994) did a survey with riders in the USA and found that 26.9% of them had an injury at least once in their horse riding experience.

More than 13% of the respondents had been hospitalised at least once in their lifetime as a result of a riding injury.

Most injuries occurred while riders were mounted on horses to perform non-jumping activities. 21.9% of the accidents involved neck or back injuries. Most of the injured riders were aged between 15 and 44 and with horse riding experience of less than 10 years. As horses can weigh approximately 1000 lbs and travel at speeds up to 30 mph, falling from a running horse can be fatal, especially when riders are stepped by the horses. The risk of injury will be increased when riders are inexperienced or the horses are young and aggressive. Helmets are useful to protect the head. Although protective vests are not effective in preventing thoracolumbar spinal fractures, it will be useful to avoid rib fractures and abdominal injury (Nelson *et al.*, 1994).

WINTER SPORTS

The major winter sports that can cause cervical spine injuries include skiing, snowmobiling, snowboarding and ice hockey. In some countries, the number of cervical injuries has increased recently due to the increase of velocity, popularity and competitiveness of these sports. In a study done by Genelin *et al.* (1994) at the Innsbruck University Hospital between 1982 and 1992, 10.9% of surgically treated spinal cases was due to participation in winter sport. 81.7% of these cases were due to skiing accidents. In a study performed by Reid and Saboe (1989), snowmobiling, tobogganing and ice hockey were found to cause almost 25% of all spinal fractures within the 7-year period of their study. Tator (1984) estimated that the number of quadriplegia cases caused by ice hockey in Canada is approximately twice that caused by American football in the USA.

OTHER SPORTS

Sports that require repetitive movements can lead to premature degeneration of the cervical spine. Chronic pain can result from hypermobility or hypomobility of the cervical joints and poor neck posture will exacerbate the problem. Acute wry neck is a common condition seen in clinical practice. It usually occurs either after a sudden, quick neck movement or after sleeping with a bad posture. The aetiology is believed to be related to facet joints dysfunction or discogenic origin but the latter is less common in young athletes.

CONCLUSION

The severity of cervical spine injury in sport varies and depends on the nature of the sport. Some of the injuries are avoidable if athletes play sensibly, following the rules of game, use proper technique and wear the appropriate protective device (e.g. helmets). Sufficient training in both muscle power and joint flexibility of the neck is equally important. Although catastrophic cervical spine injuries is apparently uncommon in Hong Kong, a systematic documentation system is required to record local sport injuries. This will be helpful in providing some figures for epidemiological study and sport injury prevention programmes in Hong Kong. Sport safety education is essential and should be started early in school. This is because travelling and studying overseas is quite popular among young people and they are likely to participate in different types of sports abroad.

In this chapter, cervical trauma related to sports has been discussed. As the method of clinical investigations, medical management and principles of treatment of these injuries are similar to those caused by other non-sport injuries, readers are advised to refer to relevant chapters in other textbooks for details. However, it is important to remember that the physical demands in different sports are not the same. A comprehensive rehabilitation programme should be designed to meet the specific flexibility and strength required by the individual athlete. Dynamic posture of the neck and sporting techniques should also be further investigated so that recurrence of neck disorders due to sports can be prevented in the future.

References:

Australian Rugby Football Union Ltd. Rugby union under 19 laws, a guide for coaches, referees and players, 1993 variations. 1993.

Bauze R.J. Experimental production of forward dislocation in the human cervical spine. J Bone Joint Surg 1978;60B:239.

Bauze R.J., Ardan G.M. Experimental production of forward dislocation in the human cervical spine. J Bone Joint Surg 1978;60B:239-45.

Blanksby B.A., Wearne F.K., Elliott B.C., Blitvich J.D. Aetiology and occurrence of diving injuries. A review of diving safety. Sports Med 1997;23:228-46.

Burstein et al. Mechanisms and pathomechanism of athletic injuries to the cervical spine. Philadelphia. Lea and Febiger 1982.

Chalmers D.J., Hume P.A., Wilson B.D. Trampolines in New Zealand: a decade of injuries. Br J Sports Med 1994;28:234-8.

Genelin A., Kathrein A., Daniaux A., Lang T., Seykora P. Schweiz Z Med
    Traumatol 1994;1:17-20.
Harries M., Williams C., Stanish W.D. and Micheli LJ. Oxford Textbook of
    Sports Medicine, Oxford Medical Publications 1994:686-97.
Johnson R.J., Lombardo J. Current Review of Sports Medicine, Current
    Medicine Philadelphia 1994:1-16.
Morrison I. Play the Game: Rugby Union, Blandford, 1993.
Nelson C. Play the Game: American Football, Blandford, 1993.
Nelson D.E., Rivara F.P., Condie C., Smith S.M. Injuries in Equestrian Sports.
    Physician Sports Med 1994;22:10:53-60.
Peterson L., Renstrom P. Sports Injuries: Their Prevention and Treatment.
    Martin Dunitz 1992:239-42
Reid D.C., Saboe L. Spine fractures in winter sports. Sports Medicine
    (Auckland) 1989;7:393-9.
Reid D.C. Sports Injury Assessment and Rehabilitation, Churchill
    Livingstone, 1992: 739-838.
Silver J.R., Gill S. Injuries of the spine sustained during rugby. Sports
    Medicine 1998;5:328-34.
Tator C.H., Edmonds V.E. National survey of spine injuries in hockey players.
    Can Med Asso J 1984;7:875-80.
Torg J.S., Quedenfeld T.C., Burstein A., Spealman A., Nichols III. National
    football head and neck injury registry: report of cervical quadriplegia,
    1971 to 1975. Am J Sports Med 1979;17:127-32.
Torg J.S. Epidemiology, biomechanics and prevention of cervical spine trauma
    resulting from athletics and recreational activities. Operative
    Techniques in Sports Med 1993;1:159-68.
Torg J.S., Sennett B., Vegso J.J., Pavlov H. Axial loading injuries to the
    middle cervical spine segment, an analysis and classification of 25
    cases. Am J Sports Med 1991a;19:6-20.
Torg J.S. Athletic Injuries to the Head, Neck and Face, Mosby Year Book
    1991b:15-27, 85-198, 338-368,438-532.

Suggested reading list:

Bloomfield J., Fricker P.A., Fitch K.D. Textbook of Science and Medicine in
    Sports, Blackwell Scientific Publications 1992:317-324.
Rao K.A. Boxing~'the sport we love to hate'. Sports Ex Inj 1995;1:124-30.
Tabor C.H., Edmonds V.E. Sports and recreation are a rising cause of spinal
    cord injury. Physician Sports Med 1986;14:157.

PART IV

Rehabilitation of Patients with Cervical Spinal Disorders

CHAPTER 12

PRINCIPLES OF NECK PAIN REHABILITATION

Thomas T.W. Chiu

INTRODUCTION

Neck pain is a common type of musculoskeletal disorder in the general population. In a nation wide healthcare survey conducted in Sweden, the prevalence of neck pain was found to be 30% (Anderson *et al.*, 1993). In Hong Kong, a household survey performed by Lau *et al.* (1996) found that the one-year prevalence rates of neck pain were 15% in men and 17% in women. Most of them are managers and professionals. Moreover, Kamwendo *et al.* (1991) and Maeda, (1977) suggested that the prevalence of neck pain is high among sedentary workers and the number is increasing. Because of the growing number of neck pain patients and the complexity of the causes of pain, the rehabilitation of neck pain patients is a challenge to therapists in this century.

CLINICAL REASONING

The fundamental requirement for successful management of neck pain is to perform an accurate physical diagnosis and a continuous evaluation of treatment outcomes. This can only be achieved with a clinical reasoning process. Clinical reasoning is the thinking of the underlying clinical practice and is the foundation of professional practice.

Without clinical reasoning, clinical practice becomes a technical operation, therapists will then just follow instructions from a superior or a decision-maker (Higgs and Jones, 1995). Jones (1992) modified the model of medical problem solving proposed by Barrows and Tamblyn (1980) and developed a model of clinical reasoning process in physical therapy. This model is illustrated in Figure 1.

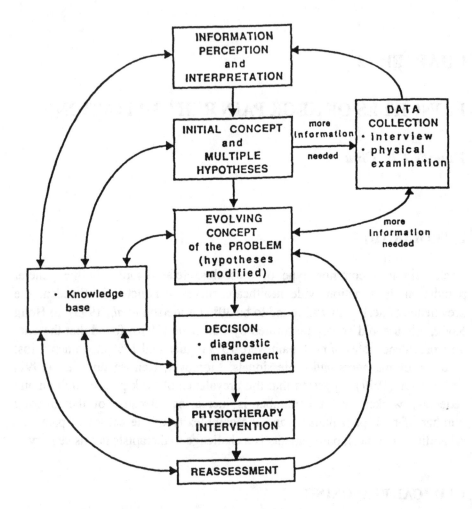

Figure 1. Model of the clinical reasoning process in physical therapy (Jones, 1992).

Clinical reasoning begins with the initial data obtained, e.g. in the management of neck pain patients, it can be a doctor's referral. Further information is then obtained through subjective examination. This information is interpreted and analysed based on the therapist's knowledge, so as to come up with hypotheses.

The initial hypothesis may be physical, psychological or socially related with or without a "diagnostic" implication. In the case of a patient with neck pain, the initial hypothesis may be, for example: "the facet joint of the right C3 to C5 levels may be affected, the neck extensor muscles are strained due to occupational needs".

Based on these initial hypotheses, specific inquiries and examinations will be made. Appropriate physical examinations can then be performed to search for supporting or negating evidence.

This hypothesis generation and testing process should be continued in order to make a physical diagnosis (i.e. to identify the sources of patient's problems) and a management plan (Jones, 1995). It must be emphasised that this clinical reasoning process must be performed continuously throughout the whole process of rehabilitation. During treatment intervention, new hypotheses may be set up. The hypothesis testing process will be further continued until the patient is discharged.

SOURCES OF NECK PAIN

Pain is defined as an unpleasant sensory and emotional experience associated with actual or potential tissue damage or an experience described in terms of such damage. Pain is a subjective perception due to mechanical and/or chemical change of body tissues. In any state of pain, the peripheral nervous system the central nervous system, the autonomic nervous system and emotional mechanisms will be involved. Therefore, anatomical, physiological and psychological factors must be considered in the planning of rehabilitation programmes for patients with neck pain.

Clinical interpretation of neck pain

There are various descriptions of pain and these descriptions may help therapists to identify the physical structures that may be injured or any underlying pathogenic process that causes pain. The sources of neck pain can be either superficial somatic, deep somatic, neurogenic, radicular, viscerogenic referred or psychogenic.

Table 1 illustrates some common types of pain described by patients and their possible pathologies and structures involved. A good understanding of the sources of neck pain is essential for the clinical reasoning process, particularly in making differential diagnoses of cervical spine disorders. It also gives therapists a rationale to choose different types of treatment and to design the management plan for patients.

Table 1. Classification of neck pain (modified from Borenstein *et al.*, 1996).

Sources of pain	Possible pathology	Description of pain
Superficial somatic (skin with subcutaneous tissue)	Cellulitis, Herpes zoster	Sharp, Burning
Deep somatic (Muscles, fascia, periosteum, ligaments, joints, vessels dura)	Muscle strain, Arthritis, Fracture, Increased venous pressure	Sharp (acute) Dull ache Boring
Radicular (spinal nerves)	Herniated vertebral disc, Foraminal stenosis	Segmental Radiating, Shooting
Neurogenic	Herpes zoster, Brachial plexopathy	Burning
Viscerogenic referred (cardiac and carotid structures)	Myocardial infraction, Carotidynis, Oesophageal spasm	Deep, Heaviness Boring Colicky
Psychogenic	Depression, Conversion reaction, Malingering	Variable

PHSYICAL IMPAIRMENTS IN THE NEURO-MUSCULOSKELETAL SYSTEM OF NECK PAIN PATIENTS

As discussed above, there are different sources of pain, therapists should be careful to find out if there are physical impairments in either articular, muscular or nervous systems of the neck. This is because these systems are closely interrelated and one may affect the others. These systems are assessed collectively with objective examinations through postural analysis, active movement test, palpation, passive accessory intervertebral movement test (PAIVM) and other specific tests, e.g. neurological test, upper limb tension tests, etc. In the following subsections, impairments in these systems will be discussed individually.

Articular system

The articular system of the cervical spine includes the atlanto-occipital joints, intervertebral joints, facet joints and uncovertebral joints between C1 and T1. However, the joints between T1 and T4 should also be assessed. Observation, active movement testing, palpation, PAIVM and passive physiological intervertebral movement test (PPIVM) are common objective examination techniques employed by therapists in assessing the articular system of patients with neck pain. A number of studies (Jull *et al.*, 1988; Sandmark and Nisell, 1995; Jull *et al.*, 1997) demonstrated that manual examination is effective to detect the presence of articular dysfunctions. There is a common misunderstanding that the presence of some hypomobility or hypermobility of the joint is diagnostic. However, this is not true as these signs can also be found in asymptomatic populations (Jull, 1986).

Jull (1997) highlighted three important elements in the manual examination of the neck. One is the perception of motion, e.g. during active movement test or PPIVM, it is important to assess the quality of movement, as well as the range. Another one is the perceived nature of tissue compliance and the reaction of tissues to applied manual stress, e.g. whether there is any abnormal end feel during PAIVM or thickening of joint capsule during palpation. The third important element is the provocation of comparable pain. These three elements are important in making clinical diagnosis of articular problems. Therapists should acquire good manual examination skills in order to avoid false positive findings caused by poor skill or handling.

Muscular system

Neck muscles are embedded with a number of proprioceptors which play a vital role in balance and postural control. Recently, the role of deep neck muscles in controlling and supporting the cervical spine has been demonstrated in a number of studies. Winters and Peles (1990) studied the interaction between neck muscles by computer modelling. They suggested that deep muscle activity was required to stiffen or stabilise the cervical spine during motion. Moreover, Mayoux-Benhamou *et al.* (1994) advocated that deep muscles of the cervical spine (longus colli and dorsal neck muscles) are important to maintain the stability of the cervical spine. They may serve as "dynamic ligaments" between vertebrae while large muscles of the cervical spine produce movement of the neck. Janda (1994) proposed three dysfunctions of muscular system, such as muscle imbalance, altered movement patterns and trigger points, should be assessed. Assessment of muscle imbalance and altered movement patterns can be performed in objective examinations. Assessment techniques include observation, deep palpation to evaluate the muscle tone, examination of the cervical spinal motion and testing of muscle tightness.

The relationship between neck pain and neck muscles has been investigated in a number of studies. In a pilot study, Hallgren *et al.* (1994) demonstrated that suboccipital muscles have been replaced by fatty tissue in patients with chronic neck pain. Barton *et al.* (1996) compared the neck muscle strength, efficiency and relaxation times between normal subjects and patients with neck pain. Their results demonstrated that all force values were significantly low in patients with neck pain. Highland *et al.* (1992) investigated the treatment effects of a specific neck exercise programme in 90 neck pain patients. Post training evaluation showed that the patients' neck strength increased significantly while their pain decreased. They also note that there was an increase of beta-endorphin level in the patients' blood serum. These results suggest that the increase of endorphin secretion may increase the patients' pain tolerance and then decrease their anxiety and tension (McArdle *et al.*, 1991). As muscle control is usually associated with pain control (Beeton and Jull, 1994; Richardson and Jull, 1995), the decrease of pain in these patients may be due to their improvement of muscle control after the exercise programme.

Nervous system

When the nerves are irritated, the nervous system can become a source of pain, e.g. entrapment of spinal nerve in a narrowed intervertebral foramen. Assessment of the nervous system is therefore necessary. The nervous system is a mechanically and physiologically continuous structure from the brain to the end terminals in the periphery. Movement of the spine and even limbs do have some implications on the biomechanics of the nervous system. In trunk flexion, the spinal canal is 5 to 9 cm longer than that in extension. In order to accommodate this change, the spinal nerve roots and meninges will then elongate and move anteriorly. In lateral flexion, the nervous system of the concave side will shorten (Berig 1978). Shacklock *et al.* (1994) proposed that regular movement of the neural tissue is necessary for optimal physiological functions. This is supported by the fact that the vascular supply of the cord is affected by spinal movement. It is therefore believed that regular movement of the neural tissue will be helpful in improving its nutrition and excretion functions. For the normal development of nerve cells, a continuous bi-directional transport and exchange of macromolecular materials is necessary. This is known as axoplasmic flow. This flow may be altered in various diseases. Biomechanical factors, e.g. stretching, torsion and compression of nerves or nerve roots, can also alter the flow. Altered axoplasmic flow is suggested to be the cause of the "double crush syndrome". Dahlin and Lundborg (1990) suggested that if a neurone is injured and its axoplasmic flow is disturbed, there will be detrimental effects on the neurone, neighbouring neurones, nerve cell bodies and their target tissues. Compression or irritation of a nerve at a site may reduce the ability of the nerve to withstand trauma (e.g. compression or irritation) at another site, making the nerve further vulnerable to trauma. For example, in a patient with chronic neck pain, an irritation of the C5 nerve root over the cervical spine may weaken the median nerve and lead to carpal tunnel syndrome in the wrist. This is supported by a number of clinical studies (Upton and McComas, 1973; Hurst *et al.*, 1985; Osterman, 1988) which demonstrated a direct relationship between carpal tunnel syndrome and cervical radiculopathy. It is clear that the mechanics and physiology of the nervous system are dynamically interrelated. Therefore, "neuropathodynamic" has been a common term to describe the association between pathomechanics and pathophysiology of neuro-disorders. As the nervous and muscular systems are very closely related, when neural tissue is irritated, they will become hypersensitive to stretching or movement and induce the responses in the muscular system. For example, it has been demonstrated that a decrease of neural extensibility in the brachial plexus is associated with an increase of muscle tension in the upper trapezius muscle (Elvey, 1979; Balster & Jull, 1997).

MANAGEMENT OF NECK PAIN PATIENTS

Having performed appropriate subjective and objective examinations, valuable information will be generated through the clinical reasoning process. This information will be used to establish the short-term management goal (e.g. to relief acute neck pain) and long-term goal (e.g. postural correction or ergonomic adaptation on work place) for patients. Then, specific treatment plans can be proposed to address the physical impairments in either the articular, muscular and/or nervous system(s). It should be noted that these treatment plans must be evaluated continuously during the treatment sessions. Modifications of the plan may be required to cope with the progression of patients' conditions.

Articular system

Articular impairment in the cervical spine can be managed by a combination of therapy methods, e.g. manipulative therapy, electrotherapy, exercise therapy and cervical traction, etc. Manipulative therapy utilised different types of mobilisation techniques (physiological movement and accessory movement) and even manipulative thrust to treat symptoms.

A number of studies demonstrated that manipulative therapy utilised both biomechanical and neurophysiological means to relieve pain and restore joint motion (Venron, 1989; Lee *et al.*, 1993; Wright, 1995). However, Nansel *et al.* (1990) reported that the increase in the range of motion provided by manipulative techniques may not last beyond 48 hours.

Therefore, any increase in joint range should be maintained by home exercise and the exercise programme should specifically cater for individual needs.

Muscular system

Good muscular support for the neck is important because the cervical spine is subject to multidirectional strain. Therefore, dysfunctions of the muscular system should be addressed as soon as possible in the rehabilitation of patients with neck pain. The basic principle is that muscle should be stretched either passively or actively if it is tight and muscles should be strengthened if it is weak.

Apart from strengthening the superficial torque producing muscles, e.g. cervical extensors, by active resisted exercise (Highland *et al.*, 1992), Jull (1997) proposed that re-education of deep cervical muscles, e.g. the deep neck flexors, and scapular girdle supporting muscles, e.g. lower trapezius and serratus anterior, should be done using isolated training method. This will provide support to the cervical spine and shoulder girdle, which is vital for successfully dealing with neck pain.

Nervous system

Therapists should be able to identify if neural tissues are involved by assessing the type of pain (e.g. sharp, shooting pain along the nerve distribution) and other signs and symptoms, such as deficit in reflex test or altered skin sensation etc. Butler (1991) proposed upper limb tension tests, a series of specific tests, to identify any abnormal mechanical tension in the median nerve, ulnar nerve and the radial nerve. He then further suggested that such abnormal tension can be addressed by the following methods:

1. Direct mobilisation of the nervous system using different techniques of the upper limb tension test or passive accessory intervertebral movements.
2. Treatment via interface and related tissue such as joints, muscles, and fascia.

3. Postural advice and ergonomic design of daily equipment, e.g. correct positioning of the keyboard will be helpful in decreasing the damage to the median nerve in regular computer users.

It should be emphasised that the articular, muscular and nervous systems are closely inter-related. For example, in neck pain patients, when the intervertebral joints are stiff, muscle tension of the upper trapezius muscle increases and neural extensibility of the brachial plexus decreases. Therefore, treatment should address all impairments in these systems. If impairments in a particular system have not been addressed properly, it will reduce the effectiveness of treatment and may lead to recurrence of problems. Apart from providing treatment in the clinic, specific exercise programmes for individual patient is very important to strengthen up the treatment effectiveness. Moreover, for successful management, advice on ergonomic for work environment, postural re-education and life-style advice should also be given accordingly.

OUTCOME MEASURES IN REHABILITATION OF NECK PAIN

There is an increasing demand for accountability in the medical system and in evidence-based practice. There is also increasing awareness of the importance of patient's perspectives, which are essential both in making medical decisions and in judging treatment results. Improvement of patients' "quality of life" is now often regarded as one of the main goals of therapy, rather than just to relieve pain or improve the range of motions. Therefore, outcomes measurement is an essential element in the rehabilitation of neck pain patients. This will be useful to maintain the standard of quality assurance and to prove the effectiveness of treatment. Outcome measurement is the evaluation of the patient's status either in terms of symptoms or functions. This should be carried out during the patient's first visit in order to establish a baseline measurement and assist the setting of treatment goals. The data obtained will be helpful in programme assessment and the final evaluation of treatment outcomes (Liebenson and Yeomans, 1997). It can also provide feedback and motivation to patients. There is a number of measurement tools in different assessment categories (e.g. pain perception, condition-specific functional disability, general health, patient satisfaction psychometrics etc.) Pain can be measured by a visual analogue scale, (Von Korff *et al.*, 1993) McGill Pain Questionnaire (Melzack, 1982) or pain diagram (Kirkaldy-Willis, 1983) etc. Unlike the case for lower back pain, measurement tools designed for the assessment of a patient's disability due to neck pain are rare in the literature.

The Neck Disability Index (Vernon and Moir, 1991) and the Northwick Park Neck Pain questionnaire (Leak *et al.*, 1994) are two measurement tools commonly employed in the clinical setting. As the format of these tools are not compatible, once the tool is chosen for outcome measurement, it should be used throughout the course of rehabilitation. Regular comparison between baseline measurements and follow up assessment results is then possible.

CONCLUSION

The first step towards successful rehabilitation of neck pain depends on appropriate identification of the physical impairments in the articular, muscular and nervous systems. This can only be achieved with a good clinical reasoning process throughout the whole course of rehabilitation. Treatment plans should address all the physical impairments. Continuous evaluation is important by using suitable outcomes measurement tools. Modifications of treatment should be made whenever necessary.

References:

Andersson H.I., Ejlertsson G., Leden I., Rosenberg C. Chronic pain in a geographically defined general population: studies of differences in age, gender, social class and pain localization. Clin J Pain 1993;9:174-82.

Balster S., Jull G. Upper trapezius muscle activity in the brachial plexus tension test in asymptomatic individuals. Manual Ther 1997;2:144-9.

Barrows H.S., Tamblyn R.M. Problem-based Learning: An Approach to Medical Education. New York, Springer 1980.

Barton P.M., Hayes K.C. Neck flexor muscle strength, efficiency, and relaxation times in normal subjects and subjects with unilateral neck pain and headache. Arch Phys Med Rehabil 1996;77:680-7.

Beeton K., Jull G.A. Effectiveness of manipulative physiotherapy in the management of cervicogenic headache: a single case study. Physiotherapy 1994;80:417-23.

Berig A. Adverse mechanical tensions in the central nervous system. Stockholm, Almqvist and Wisksell 1978.

Borenstein D.G., Wiesel S.W., Boden S.D. Neck Pain Medical Diagnosis and Comprehensive Management. Saunders 1996:33-63.

Butler D. Mobilisation of the Nervous System. Melbourne, Churchill Livingstone 1991.

Dahlin L.B., Lundborg G. The neurone and its response to peripheral nerve compression. J Hand Surg 1990;15B:5-10.

Elvey R.L. In Chapter 3: Brachial plexus tension test and the pathoanatomical origin of arm pain. In: Glasgow EF, Twomey LT eds, Aspects of Manipulative Therapy. First edition, Melbourne, Lincoln Institute of Health Sciences 1979;3:105-10.

Hallgren R.C., Greenman P.E., Rechtien J.J. Atrophy of suboccipital muscles in patient with chronic pain: a pilot study. J Am Osteop Assoc 1994;94:1032-9.

Higgs J., Jones M. Clinical reasoning in the Health Professions. London, Butterworth-Heinemann 1995.

Highalnd T.R., Dreisinger T.E., Vie L.L., Russell G.S. Changes in Isometric strength and range of motion of the isolated cervical spine after eight weeks of clinical rehabilitation. Spine 1992;17[Suppl]:S77-82.

Hurst L.C., Wiessberg D., Caroll R.E. The relationship of the double crush to carpal tunnel syndrome (analysis of 1000 cases of carpal tunnel syndrome). J Hand Surg 1985;19B:202-4.

Janda V. Muscles and motor control in cervicogenic disorders: assessment and management. In: Grant R ed, Physical Therapy of the Cervical and Thoracic Spine. Churchill Livingstone 1994:195-216.

Jones M.A. Clinical reasoning and Pain. Manual Ther 1995;1:17-24.

Jones M.A. Clinical reasoning in manual therapy. Phys Ther 1992;72:875-84.

Jull G.A., Bogduk N., Marsland A. The accuracy of manual diagnosis for cervical zygapophyseal joint pain syndromes. Med J Aust 1988;148:233-6.

Jull G.A. Clinical observation of upper limb mobility. In: Grieve GP ed, Modern Manual Therapy of the Vertebral Column. Edinburgh, Churchill Livingstone 1986:315-21.

Jull G.A. Management of cervical headache. Manual Ther 1997;2:182-90.

Kamwendo K., Linton S.J., Moritz U. Neck and shoulder disorders in medical secretaries. Part I: Pain prevalence and risk factors. Scand J Rehab Med 1991;23:127-33.

Kirkaldy-Willis W.H. Managing low back pain. New York, Churchill Livingstone 1983.

Lau E.M.C., Sham A., Wong K.C. The prevalence of and risk factors for neck pain in Hong Kong Chinese. J Public Health Med 1996;18:396-9.

Leak A.M., Cooper J., Dyer S., Williams K.A., Turner-Stroke L., Frank A.O. The Northwick Park Neck Pain Questionnaire, devised to measure neck pain and disability. Br J Rheumat 1994;33:469-74.

Lee M., Latimer J., Maher C. Manipulation: investigation of a proposed mechanism. Clin Biomech 1993;8:302-6.

Liebensen C., Yeomans S. Outcomes assessment in musculoskeletal medicine. Manual Ther 1997;2:67-74.

Maeda K. Occupational cervicobrachial disorder and its causative factors. J Hum Ergol 1977:193-202.

Mayoux-Benhamou M.A., Revel M., Vallee C., Roudier R., Barbet J.P., Bargy F. Longus colli has a postural function on cervical curvature. Surg Radiol Anat 1994;16:367-71.

McArdle W.D., Katch F.I., Kath V.L. Exercise Physiology energy, nutrition, and human performance. Lea and Febiger 1991:384-417.

Melzack R. Pain measurement and assessment. New York, Raven Press 1982.

Nansel D., Peneff A., Cremata E., Carlson J. Time course consideration for the effect of unilateral lower cervical adjustments with respect to the amelioration of cervical lateral-flexion passive end-range asymmetry. J Manip Physiol Ther 1990;13:297-304.

Osterman A. The double crush syndrome. Orthop Clin North Am 1988;19:147-55.

Richardson C.A., Jull G.A. Muscle control-pain control. What exercise would you prescribe? Manual Ther 1995;1:2-10.

Sandmark H., Nisell R. Validity of five common manual neck pain provocating tests. Scand J Rehab Med 1995;27:131-6.

Shacklock M., Butler D., Salter H. The dynamic cervical nervous system: structure and clinical neurobiomechanics. In: Boyling J.D. and Palastanga N. eds, Grieve's Modern Manual therapy of the Vertebral column, Second edition, Edinburgh, Churchill Livingstone 1994:21-38.

Upton R., McComas A. The double crush in nerve entrapment syndrome. Lancet 1973;18:359-61.

Vernon H., Mior S. The neck disability index: A study of reliability and validity. J Manip Physiol Ther 1991;14:409-15.

Vernon H. Exploring the effect of a spinal manipulation on plasma beta-endorphin levels in normal men. Spine 1989;14:1272-3.

Von Korff M., Deyo R.A., Cherkin D., Barlow W. Back pain in primary care: outcomes at one year. Spine 1993;18:855-62.

Winters J.M., Peles J.D. Neck muscle activity and 3-D head kinematics during quasi-static and dynamic tracking movements. In: Winters J.M., Woo SL-Y. eds, Multiple Muscle System: Biomechanics and Movement Organisation. New York, Springer-Verlag, 1990:461-80.

Wright A. Hypoalgesia post-manipulative therapy: a review of a potential neurophysiological mechanism. Manual Ther 1995;1:11-6

CHAPTER 13

ELECTROTHERAPY FOR CERVICAL SPINAL DISORDERS

Grace P.Y. Szeto

INTRODUCTION

Electrophysical agents are frequently used by physiotherapists to treat musculoskeletal conditions. The projected physiological effects include increased blood flow and tissue temperature, increased metabolism, reduced muscle spasm and reduction in pain (Low and Reed, 1994; Michlovitz, 1990a; Kitchen and Bazin, 1996). While more scientific research is required to substantiate all of these mechanisms, the basic physiological effects of electrophysical agents are well recognised and accepted by the clinical communities. With reference to disorders in the cervical region, the goal of treatment with electrophysical agents is not to alter primary pathological changes in skeletal tissues. As in other conditions, the effects of electrotherapy are mainly directed at the soft tissues or inflammatory changes in the soft tissues. The clinical conditions in the cervical spine that are commonly treated with electrophysical therapeutic agents include:

(1) cervical spondylosis,
(2) facet joint dysfunctions,
(3) soft tissue problems, e.g. tightness, spasm, adhesions, weakness,
(4) cervicogenic headaches and
(5) nerve root irritation or compression.

The objective of this chapter is not to provide a comprehensive step-by-step instruction manual on the theories and methods of application of all electrotherapy modalities. Based on the author's clinical experience and on review of research evidence, it aims to provide readers with a set of useful guidelines in the application of these modalities to provide effective treatment for the common conditions of the cervical spine.

PHYSIOTHERAPY ASSESSMENT

Before planning a physiotherapy treatment programme, a complete and thorough assessment must be performed. The findings of the assessment will form the basis from which the clinical reasoning process can develop. From the assessment, the physiotherapist can identify and prioritise the patient's problems and formulate the treatment plan. Then the therapist can consider carefully which modality can achieve the treatment goals most effectively and efficiently. The use of electrophysical agents is often an integral part of the physiotherapy management plan. Its application must be complimentary with other treatment, including exercise prescription, manual therapy and functional rehabilitation.

SELECTING APPROPRIATE ELECTROPHYSICAL AGENTS

As the number and the variety of electrophysical agents are growing, the physiotherapist is often faced with the dilemma of selecting an appropriate modality for their patients, out of many modalities available. This is particularly crucial in the current socioeconomic climate, as medical and allied health professionals are expected to justify the efficacy and cost-effectiveness of their services. There are a number of important factors that a physiotherapist must consider in selecting an appropriate electrophysical modality for treatment:

(1) patient's problem(s) and treatment goals;
(2) stage of injury or disease, e.g. acute, sub-acute or chronic, presence and nature of any swelling or active inflammation must be noted;
(3) specific therapeutic effects desired, e.g. pain relief, muscle relaxation, increasing tissue extensibility, increasing blood flow, promoting resolution of inflammation, reducing oedema, muscle re-education and so on;
(4) dimensions of treatment area, e.g. shape, size and contour of body region to be treated;
(5) tissue composition in the treatment area, e.g. the thickness of different tissue layers including fatty tissues, the location and extent of vascular and neural tissues;
(6) depth of penetration required for therapeutic effects, compared to what the modality can produce;
(7) contra-indications to treatment with different modalities, e.g. these include adverse skin conditions or reactions, unstable cardiovascular conditions, cardiac pacemakers, active tumours, and the presence of metal;

(8) precautions to be taken to ensure safety during treatment and no adverse reaction afterwards;

(9) availability of equipment, space and time.

In treating cervical spinal problems, it is often necessary to extend the treatment areas into the suboccipital region, the scapular region or the upper thoracic region, as the muscles and ligaments of the cervical spine often span over these areas. It is also important to recognise specific problems with individual patients, as the labelling of a diagnosis or "syndrome" does not always mean that the patients will exhibit the same signs and symptoms associated with that diagnosis, nor that the patients will always respond in the same way to treatment. The electrotherapy modalities, including superficial thermal agents, deep thermal agents, cryotherapy, ultra-sound, electrical stimulation and laser, will be discussed in the following subsections.

1. Superficial thermal agents

In physiotherapy, superficial thermal agents commonly used include hot packs, wax baths, infra-red light and whirlpools. The physiological effects of these modalities are mainly: (i) to increase local tissue temperature and blood flow, (ii) to induce muscle relaxation and (iii) to increase tissue extensibility (Michlovitz, 1990a; Low and Reed, 1994).

Conductive and convection heating can also produce temperature increase in local tissue (Collins, 1996; Michlovitz, 1990). For treatment of cervical spine disorders, hot packs and infra-red light may be more appropriate to produce superficial thermal effects, while wax and whirlpools are usually prescribed for the treatment of peripheral conditions.

Hot packs and infra-red light are both relatively safe and contra-indications due to their usage are rare. The advantage of using hot packs lies in its ease of application and ability to mould over the treatment surface. There are different shapes and sizes of hot packs. In particular, "cervical" hot packs can be easily wrapped around the neck, providing heat to both the lateral and posterior surfaces of the neck. It can also be placed flat under the patient's neck and both shoulders. Patients should not experience extreme heat on the skin immediately, but the heat should build up during the treatment. Care must be taken to ensure that the towelling covers are sufficient. Otherwise, there may be a danger of causing burns.

The general guidelines for producing local temperature increases using heat modalities have been described by several authors (Lehman and deLateur, 1982; Michlovitz, 1990a; McMeekan, 1994; Low and Reed, 1994). Generally it is thought that tissue temperature needs to rise above 40°C up to 45°C for hyperemia (increased blood flow) to occur. With vasodilatation, the increased blood flow may bring more of the "cooler" blood to the region and thereby dissipate some of the heat generated in the local tissues. Thus, it is often difficult to estimate the exact extent of tissue temperature change and the duration of such changes.

Increase in skin blood flow may occur via three mechanisms: (1) axon reflex, (2) release of chemical mediators secondary to temperature elevation, (3) local spinal cord reflexes (Michlovitz, 1990a). The physiological mechanisms by which heating the local tissues can elicit pain relief are summarised in Figure 1.

Infra-red therapy is one of the superficial thermal agents that has become less commonly used in the physiotherapy department. However, there seems to be increasing popularity of this modality as a form of home treatment. Some of the commercially available infra-red lamps are quite compact and can be easily applied.

When patients seek advice from the physiotherapists on the use of these lamps at home, it is important to teach patients the proper methods and precautionary measures, in order to achieve effective results and avoid causing skin burn. These include applying the lamp at an appropriate distance, setting a safe intensity level of the lamp, monitoring skin condition for erythema and moisture and checking if the skin has a normal sensation.

2. Deep thermal agents

In physiotherapy, deep thermal agents usually refer to shortwave diathermy and microwave diathermy. Both are high frequency currents, which can generate electromagnetic radiation. For shortwave diathermy, the frequency at 27.12 MHz is most widely used in almost all types of shortwave machines.

Generally, shortwave is much more commonly used than microwave by therapists according to published surveys (Lindsay *et al.*, 1990; Pope *et al.*, 1995). In the cervical spine, shortwave is commonly applied using a coplanar method (Figure 2). In this method, two flexible pads or two disc electrodes will be used to produce an electric field along the posterior musculature and soft tissues, without heating the anterior vascular and neural structures of the cervical spine.

The heat produced by shortwave is dependent on the electromagnetic field set up in the tissues, which is determined by tissue conductivity (Scott, 1996). Tissues containing high water content, such as muscles and blood vessels, will be heated up more quickly than fatty tissue and bone using shortwave diathermy (Low and Reed, 1994).

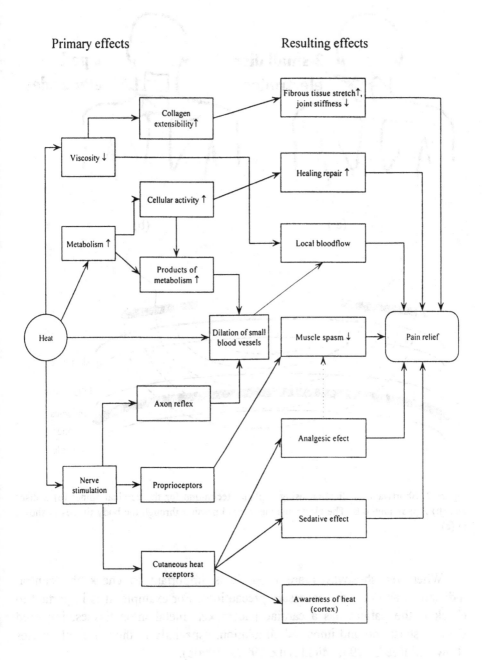

Figure 1. Physiological events produced by heating local tissues
(adapted from Low and Reed, 1994:199)

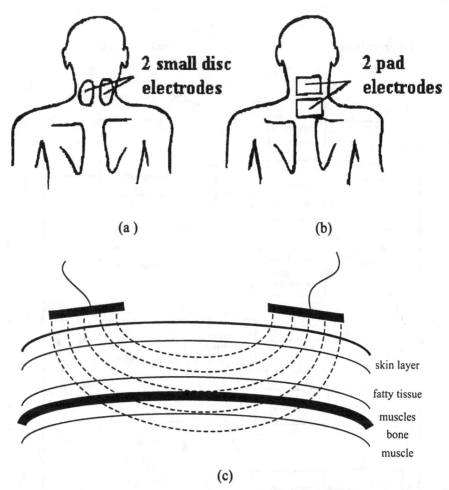

(a)   **(b)**

2 small disc electrodes

2 pad electrodes

skin layer

fatty tissue

muscles

bone

muscle

(c)

Figure 2. Shortwave application using coplanar technique for the cervical spine: (a) 2 discs and (b) 2 pads methods. The electromagnetic field passing through the body tissues is shown in (c).

Whenever shortwaves are used, it is important to check the contra-indications and take the necessary precautions. For example, it is important to check if the patient has a cardiac pacemaker, metal in/on tissues, impaired thermal sensation and impaired circulation, especially in the vertebral arteries (Low and Reed, 1994; Michlovitz, 1990a; 1990b).

Microwave (MW) diathermy is another form of electromagnetic energy that can produce a deep heating effect and increase blood flow (McMeekan, 1994). However, it has never been as popular as shortwave in clinical practice. The major concern with MW irradiation is the possibility of overheating the fatty tissues and tissue boundaries, as microwaves are concentrated in these regions due to refraction and reflection (Kloth and Ziskin, 1990).

Shortwave diathermy can be applied in either continuous or pulsed modes. Machines, such as the Curapuls, usually provide options of continuous and pulsed modes and a number of pre-set pulse frequencies. The pulsed mode will give minimal thermal effects and the patient will hardly feel any heating sensation.

Pulsed shortwave is considered to be a form of high-frequency "pulsed electromagnetic energy" (PEME), which can also be applied in the form of low-frequency magnetic fields. The low frequency field is usually set at frequencies of less than 100Hz, and its effects have been suggested to be similar to those of the pulsed shortwave (Low and Reed, 1994). Its advantages lie in its ease of application and relatively few contra-indications involved. Clinically, there has been increasing applications of this modality in treating both acute and chronic pain, as well as soft tissue injuries. It has been suggested that PEME may promote healing by repolarising damaged cells through reactivating the sodium pump at the cell membrane during the inflammatory stage (Kloth and Ziskin, 1990). McMeekan (1992) studied the tissue temperature and blood flow changes in human forearm muscles following magnetic field therapy. No significant increase in blood flow was found. The electro-magnetic field has been suggested to be able to promote tissue healing and resolution of inflammation (Low and Reed, 1994).

3. Cryotherapy

In the treatment of cervical spinal disorders, ice therapy is not used as commonly as heat. This is because heat is relatively effective for relieving muscle tightness and joint stiffness. However, ice therapy will be useful when there is acute muscle spasm as in acute wry neck. In this case, ice packs may be an appropriate choice to produce a sedative effect on the sensory nerves and to relieve muscle spasm (Michlovitz, 1990b).

4. Ultrasound

Ultra-sound therapy is frequently used in physiotherapy treatment for soft tissue injuries. The main physiological effects of ultrasound include acoustic streaming, cavitation and micromassage (Kitchen and Partridge, 1990; Fyfe and Bullock, 1985), which are produced by mechanical vibrations rather than heat effects. These mechanical effects can facilitate the diffusion of calcium ions across the cell membrane and stimulate the movements of tissue fluids, which will ultimately promote the resolution of the inflammatory process (Fyfe and Bullock, 1985; Dyson 1987).

Ultrasound is commonly used for treating musculoskeletal disorders in the cervical and scapular regions. As the ultrasound head comes in different sizes, the sound waves can be positioned directly over the target soft tissues, it can treat the muscles of the cervical spine without affecting sensitive neurovascular structures. For example, using a small treatment head, an ultra-sound beam can be directed to treat either localised tender spots or the whole length of sternocleidomastoids and scalene muscles.

When ultrasound is applied, therapists are required to determine a number of treatment parameters, including frequency of the ultra-sound, area of insonation, power, intensity (spatial average, temporal average, spatial peak, temporal peak), mark/space ratio (duty cycle), time of irradiation and beam non-uniformity ratio (Kitchen and Partridge, 1990; Young 1996). The projected therapeutic effects of ultrasound are promoting blood flow, mobilising adhesions of soft tissues and increasing tissue extensibility (Dyson, 1987). It has been suggested that ultrasound can also reduce bruising and swelling effects in the acute phase of soft tissue inflammation (Fyfe and Chahl, 1982). Enwemeka *et al.* (1990) reported that ultrasound can increase tensile strength and elasticity in injured tendons, even at very low intensities (0.5 w/cm^2 spatial average). These reports suggest that ultra-sound will be useful to increase the extensibility of soft tissues in the cervical and scapular regions.

5. Electrical Stimulation

Electrical stimulation is often used to treat pain, inflammation and/or tightness in the soft tissues in patients with cervical spinal disorders. The most common types of electrical stimulation modalities are transcutaneous electrical nerve stimulation (TENS), interferential therapy (IFT) and high voltage galvanic stimulation (HVG). As some of the current formats in neuromuscular electrical stimulation (NMES) or functional electrical stimulation (FES) are more useful for muscle re-education or strength training, they may not be appropriate for cervicogenic problems. However, when muscle weakness or atrophy has been caused by nerve entrapment or compression, electrical stimulation (faradic or interrupted direct current) will be useful to elicit muscle contraction.

In the last two decades, the pain relieving effects of TENS have been studied extensively, especially for chronic pain. Several comprehensive review papers have been published to provide overviews in this area of research (Robinson, 1996; Roche and Wright, 1990; Oosterwijk *et al.*, 1994; Walsh, 1997). Generally, TENS is commonly applied in three modes: (1) conventional TENS, (2) acupuncture-like TENS and (3) brief intense TENS (Gersh, 1992).

Conventional TENS is usually applied for several hours with a high frequency (10-300 Hz) and low intensity current (Mannheimer and Lampe, 1984). Acupuncture-like TENS involves a low frequency current (1-10Hz) but with high current intensities. It is only applied for a short period of time. Brief intense TENS involves the application of noxious levels of stimulation at relatively high frequencies (50-100Hz) for pain control (Robinson, 1996). This approach is similar to the concept of "painful stimulation" in other electrical stimulation modalities, such as interferential therapy, whereby a high-intensity current is delivered to the area of pain and/or the trigger points (De Domenico, 1987).

IFT is another popular modality used in physiotherapy to treat acute and chronic pain, although there have not been many studies specifically focusing on the use of this form of current to prove its pain relieving effects. Stephenson and Johnson (1995) examined the effects of interferential therapy on experimentally induced pain. They reported a significant increase in pain threshold and tolerance in subjects who had received interferential therapy. The advantage of the interferential current format lies in its comfort level due to the reduction of effective skin resistance produced by the medium frequency currents. IFT basically consists of a carrier frequency usually in the range of 4000 to 4100 Hz and the blending of the two currents produces an amplitude modulated current (De Domenico, 1987). The beat frequency of the resultant current is usually within the low frequency range which is able to produce sensory and motor nerve stimulation. Because of these characteristics, IFT can be used to treat pain, muscle re-education, as well as oedema in acute or chronic inflammation. In the cervical and upper thoracic regions, IFT can be applied by using the suction cup electrodes or the rubber pad electrodes to facilitate muscle relaxation and pain relief.

HVG is another type of current used in physiotherapy. It involves the application of a direct current with twin-spiked pulses delivered by a high voltage (300-500V) for a very short duration. It is believed that such high voltage currents can penetrate more deeply down to the tissues. In clinical practice, HVG has been used for the treatment of pain, muscle re-education, as well as reduction of oedema (Kahn, 1994; Selkowitz, 1989; Quirion-De Girardi et al., 1984).

In recent years, microcurrent has been gradually adopted as another form of electrical stimulation for pain relief, as well as for wound healing. It has been proposed that microcurrents can promote tissue healing and repair (Picker, 1988a; 1988b; Watson, 1996) because this type of low intensity stimulation (in terms of microamperes) is similar to the "natural" bioelectric current in our body. Although a number of research studies support the claim that microcurrent can promote wound healing, there is little evidence to show that it has pain relieving effects. In fact, other than the TENS research, there has only been a handful of studies done in the past to substantiate the claims of the therapeutic effects of the various electrical stimulators. Although there has been a significant increase in research studies related to electrical stimulation, no conclusive evidence has shown which types of current are more effective than others to generate muscle contraction, to reduce pain or to produce muscle relaxation. McMeekan (1995) has suggested that the pulse shape and waveform of the applied current are not critical, as long as the pulse charge (product of intensity and pulse duration) is adequate to stimulate sensory and motor nerves. The mechanisms by which electrical stimulation can activate various nerve fibres are summarised in Figure 3. In fact, many textbooks have grouped various types of currents together under the heading of "electrical stimulation", "transcutaneous nerve stimulation" or "neuromuscular electrical simulation" (Low and Reed, 1994; Kitchen and Bazin, 1996; Gersh, 1992). A few general principles should be noted when using electrical stimulation modalities and they are listed as follows:

1. The combination of pulse shape, duration and intensity will affect the perception of comfort and penetration of the current into deeper tissues. Other factors, such as acute or chronic nature of the pain, size of area, tissue composition and individual preference or sensitivity, should be taken into consideration when selecting stimulus parameters.

2. The intensity of stimulation should be set at the patient's maximum tolerance, which is commonly described as the "highest comfortable tingling paraesthesia without muscle contraction" (Kloth, 1992). In the case of acute pain, muscle contraction or motor nerve activation is usually not desired. In sub-acute or chronic pain, mild rhythmical muscle contraction can be very effective in reducing pain and promoting muscle relaxation. Figure 4 is a summary of guidelines for selecting treatment parameters in various electrical stimulation agents.

3. Electrode placement is crucial for any form of electrical stimulation (Alon, 1987; Kloth, 1992; McMeekan, 1995; De Domenico, 1987). The size of the electrode used is also very important and electrodes should cover most of the treatment area. When electrical stimulation is employed to treat pain, electrodes can be placed either over the area where the pain is located or within the dermatome distribution, or at any localised tenderness points, trigger points or acupuncture points. The selection of the electrode type, size and placement should be based on the physical assessment and the clinical reasoning process (see Figure 4).

4. In order to avoid the accommodation effect of nerve fibres, some form of current modulation is desirable. However, the choice of modulation is dependent of the functions available with different stimulators. For

example, IFT current is already amplitude modulated, but some of the models also offer options of frequency modulation, vector sweep and others.

5. In all forms of electrical stimulation treatment, the main contra-indications are the presence of cardiac pacemakers, impaired circulatory problems such as thrombosis or hemorrhage problems, unstable cardiac rhythms, open wounds and pregnancy (Gersh, 1992; Low and Reed, 1994).

Electrical stimulation can be combined with ultra-sound or heat and this is in fact quite a common practice used by physiotherapists. The proposed effect is that when the two modalities are combined together, it will further enhance the increase in blood flow and/or pain relief. However, there is very little research evidence to substantiate this claim.

In recent years, stimulation of trigger points and acupuncture points have also become a common treatment approach in pain management (Melzack, 1981). This form of stimulation can be performed using point electrodes of IFT or HVG machines, or by using the probe in microcurrent therapy. Instead of using electrical stimulation to treat pain, lasers can also be used to irradiate a small localised area such as an acupuncture point. Travell and Simons (1983) have mapped out the trigger points for most of the body muscles. In cervical spine disorders, patients often exhibit tightness in trapezius and levator scapulae muscles. Using the point stimulation method, lasers can be applied at the trigger points for these muscles or specific acupuncture points to relieve symptoms. Advocates for both approaches have claimed that these treatment methods are effective. However, only a few studies have compared the treatment effects among these methods.

6. Laser therapy

Low level laser therapy (LLLT) is the application of low-output (<500mW) lasers and monochromatic superluminous diodes for the treatment of disease and injury with a dosages less than 35 J/cm^2 (Laakso *et al.*, 1993). In physiotherapy, LLLT has been used to promote wound healing, as well as to treat pain and soft tissue inflammation.

Baxter (1996) suggested that laser therapy can be applied over cervical nerve roots, brachial plexus or peripheral nerves such as median, ulnar or radial nerves where the nerves are relatively superficial. Lasers can also be used as an alternative of inserting needles at acupuncture points in treating pain. Unlike other treatment, acute soft tissue injuries can be immediately treated by laser. It has been proposed that lasers will be helpful in resolving inflammation and promoting healing (Baxter, 1996).

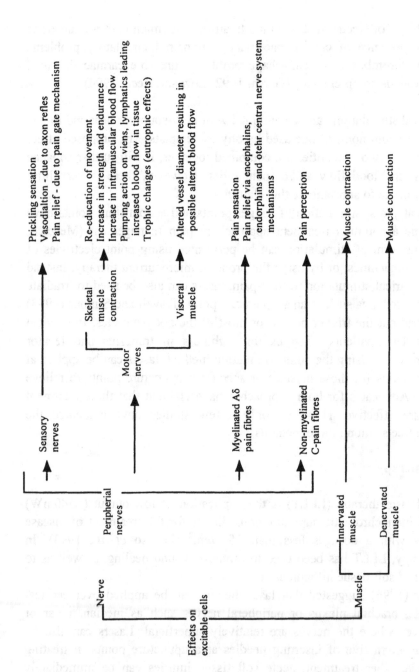

Figure 3. Effects of electrical stimulation in activating peripheral nerve fibres (adapted from Low and Reed 1994:85).

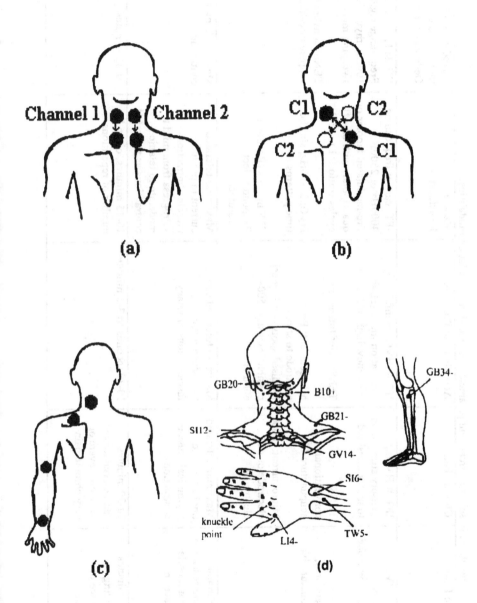

Figure 4. Electrode placement options for electrical stimulation of the cervical spine; (a) 2 channels along the erector spinae, (b) 2 channels in a cross-fire pattern, (c) electrodes placed along dermatome distribution of pain or (d) appropriate acupuncture points.

Table 1. Summary table of guidelines in selecting treatment parameters in electrical stimulation modalities.

	Acute Pain	Chronic Pain	Acute Painful Procedure	Muscle Re-education	Mixed sensory and motor problems/Oedema control
Suitable Modes of Electrical Stimulation	IFT & HVG: Sensory stimulation mode TENS: conventional, acupuncture-like	IFT & HVG: Sensory stimulation to motor threshold TENS: conventional, acupuncture-like Microcurrent: probe electrode or pad electrodes	IFT & HVG: Painful stimulation mode (High frequency, high intensity) TENS: Brief Intense mode Microcurrent: Probe electrode to stimulate localised spots – at highest possible intensity (500-600uA)	IFT: carrier freq. can be 4000Hz or 2500Hz Pre-modulated bipolar or quadripolar, with on-off cycles (ratio 1:1 to 1:4) HVG: 25-50Hz, similar time patterns FES models (Respond II, Respond Select, Neurotech)	IFT & HVG: Larger Freq. range e.g.0-100Hz, rhythmical sweeping mode TENS: conventional or acupuncture-like
Progress Amplitude to produce:	Comfortable tingling sensation without muscle contraction	Maximum tolerated tingling + mild rhythmical muscle contractions	Maximum tolerated current to produce muscle fasciculations or tetany	Maximum tolerated current to produce muscle contractions - Progress from mild to moderate to tetanic contractions as tolerated	Max. tol. Tingling and contractions
Treatment Duration	10-20 minutes depending on tolerance of patient	20-30 minutes can be even longer for more severe or very chronic pain	10-30 seconds to 3-5 minutes	10-15 minutes, or go by number of repetitions	20-45 minutes

COMBINING DIFFERENT MODALITIES IN THE SAME TREATMENT

It is common clinical practice to use more than one electrophysical modality in the same treatment session. For example, in treating an acute injury like acute wry-neck, acute whiplash or muscle strain, ice may be used followed by ultra-sound therapy, as well as manual mobilisation techniques. Although both ice therapy and ultrasound can stimulate blood flow and facilitate muscle relaxation, ultrasound is the sole agent providing mechanical vibratory effects. Hence, some modalities can be combined quite appropriately as some of the physiological effects are common, while other effects may be more specific to certain modalities.

However, in some situations, combining modalities may be redundant. For example, it is senseless to combine shortwave with microwave, or even shortwave with hot pack.

In cases where the same multiple areas are treated, it may be necessary to use more than one form of heat modality. There has also been a common practice to use hot packs and electrical stimulation concurrently. The heat is believed to facilitate the penetration of electrical current by reducing skin impedance. Patients have reported that this combination of treatment is helpful in relieving pain and promoting muscle relaxation.

The latest models of electrical stimulators often provide a combined therapy mode in which electrical current and ultrasound can be simultaneously delivered to patients using the same ultrasound treatment head. Again, the positive benefits of such treatment are mainly anecdotal and there has been very little research evidence to support this type of approach. One recent study (Lee *et al.*, 1997), however, has shown that the range of movement in the cervical spine increased significantly in patients who were treated with combined electrical stimulation and ultra-sound therapy, as compared with those who were treated with the two modalities separately.

The guideline for selecting the right modality is related to the evaluation of the treatment effects. Therapists should always evaluate the treatment results immediately after the application of each electrophysical modality. It can be done simply by observing muscle activity, assessing the range of movement or evaluating subjective complaints. This evaluation is helpful in checking whether the treatment has already produced the therapeutic effects as planned. It will also assist therapists to plan for the progression of treatment.

SUMMARY

The use of electrophysical agents is an integral part of physiotherapy management in musculoskeletal conditions. In selecting an appropriate modality for patients, therapists should consider the assessment results, the pathophysiology of the disorders and the desired therapeutic effects. Safety issues and the patient's comfort should be of primary concern to the therapist. Factors, such as the size, shape, condition and composition of body structure can often affect the penetration depth or the spread of therapeutic effects. Therapists should also consider how the application of electrotherapy can complement with the rest of the treatment programme to achieve optimal benefits for the patients. For evidence-based practice, extensive clinical research is required to substantiate the therapeutic effects of electrotherapy. This is particularly true in the clinical treatment of cervical spinal conditions.

References:

Alon G. Principles of electrical stimulation. In Nelson R.M. and Currier D.P. eds, Clinical Electrotherapy. Norwalk: Appleton & Lange 1987:29-80.

Baxter D. Low level laser therapy. In Kitchen S and Bazin S ed, Clayton's Electrotherapy 10th edition, London, Philadelphia, Toronto, Sydney, Tokyo, WB Saunders Company Ltd. 1996:197-217.

Collins K. Thermal effects. In Kitchen S. and Bazin S. eds, Clayton's Electrotherapy 10th edition. London, WB Saunders Company Ltd 1996:93-109.

De Domenico G. New dimensions in interferential therapy. A theoretical & clinical guide. Lindfield, NSW, Reid Medical Books 1987.

Dyson M. Mechanisms involved in therapeutic ultra-sound, Physiotherapy 1987;73: 116-20.

Enwemeka C.S., Rodriguez O., Mendosa S. The biomechanical effects of low-intensity ultra-sound on healing tendons. Ultra-sound Med Bio 1990;16:801-7.

Fyfe M.C., Buollock M.I. Therapeutic ultra-sound: some historical background and development in knowledge of its effect on healing. Aust J Physiotherapy 1985;31:220-4.

Fyfe M.C., Chahl L.A. Mast cell degranulation: A possible mechanism of action of therapeutic ultra-sound. Ultra-sound Med Bio 1982;8(Suppl I):62.

Gersh M.R. Transcutaneous Electrical Nerve Stimulation (TENS) for management of pain and sensory pathology. In Gersh MR ed,

Electrotherapy in Rehabilitation. Philadelphia: F.A. Davis Company 1992:149-96.

Kahn J. Principles and Practice of Electrotherapy, Third edition, NewYork, Churchill Livingstone 1994.

Kitchen S.S., Bazin S. Clayton's Electrotherapy. 10th edition, London. W.B. Saunders Company 1996.

Kitchen S.S., Partridge C.J. A review of therapeutic ultra-sound, Physiotherapy 1990;76:593-600.

Kloth L.C., Ziskin M.C. Diathermy and pulsed electromagnetic fields. In Michlovitz S.L. ed., Thermal Agents in Rehabilitation, Second edition, Philadelphia, F.A. Davis Company 1990.

Kloth LC. Electrotherapeutic alternatives for the treatment of pain. In Gersh MR ed, Electrotherapy in Rehabilitation. Philadelphia, F.A. Davis Company 1992:197-217.

Laakso L., Richardson C., Cramond T. Factors affecting low level laser therapy, Aust J Physiotherapy 1993;39:95-9.

Lee J.C., Lin D.T., Hong C.Z. The effectiveness of simultaneous thermotherapy with ultrasound and electrotherapy with combined AC and DC current on the immediate pain relief of myofascial trigger points, J Musculoskeletal Pain 1997;5:81-90.

Lehman J.F., de Lateur B.J. Therapeutic heat. In Lehman JK ed, Therapeutic Heat and Cold. Baltimore, Williams & Wilkins 1982:404-562.

Lindsay D., Dearness J., Richardson C., Chapman A., Cuskelly G. A survey of electromodality usage in private physiotherapy practices, Aust J Physiotherapy 1990;36:249-56.

Low J., Reed A (1994). Electrotherapy Explained: Principles and practice, Second edition, Oxford, Butterworth Heinemann 1994.

Mannheimer J.S., Lampe G.N. Clinical Transcutaneous Electrical Nerve Stimulation. Philadelphia, F.A. Davis Company Ltd 1984.

McMeekan J. Electrotherapy. In Zuluaga M., Briggs C., Carlisle J., McDonald V., McMeekan J., Nickson W., Oddy P., Wilson D. eds, Sports Physiotherapy, Applied science and practice. Melbourne: Churchill Livingstone 1995:233-44.

McMeekan J. Magnetic fields: effects on blood flow in human subjects, Physiotherapy Theory and Practice 1992;8:3-9.

McMeekan J. Tissue temperature and blood flow: A research based overview of electrophysical modalities. Aust J Physiotherapy 1994;40:49-57.

Melzack R. Myofascial trigger points: relation to acupuncture and mechanisms of pain. Arch Phys Med Rehab 1981;62:114-7.

Michlovitz S.L. Biophysical principles of heating and superficial heating agents. In Michlovitz S.L. ed, Thermal Agents in Rehabilitation Second edition, Philadelphia, F.A. Davis Company 1990a:88-106.

Michlovitz S.L. Cryotherapy. In Michlovitz S.L. ed, Thermal Agents in Rehabilitation. Second edition, Philadelphia, F.A. Davis Company 1990b:63-87.

Oosterwijk R.F.A., Meyler W.J., Henley E.J., Scheer S.S., Tannenbaum J. Pain control with TENS and team nerve stimulators: a review. Crit Rev Phys Rehab Med 1994;6:219-58.

Picker R.I. Low-volt pulsed microamp stimulation Part I, Clin Management 1988a;9:10-4.

Picker R.I. Low-volt pulsed microamp stimulation Part II, Clin Management 1988b;9:28-33.

Pope G.D., Mockett S.P., Wright J.P. A survey of electrotherapeutic modalities: ownership and use in the NHS in England. Physiotherapy 1995;81:82-91.

Quirion-De Girardi C., Seaborne D., Savard-Goulet F., W-Nieto M., Lambert J.L. The analgesic effect of high voltage galvanic stimulation combined with ultrasound in the treatment of low back pain: a one-group pretest/post-test study, Physiotherapy Can 1984;36:327-33.

Robinson A.J. Transcutaneous Electrical Nerve Stimulation for the control of pain in musculoskeletal disorders, J Orthop Sports Phys Ther 1996;24:208-26.

Roche P.A., Wright A. An investigation into the value of transcutaneous electrical nerve stimulation (TENS) for arthritic pain, Physiotherapy Theory and Practice 1990;6:25-33.

Scott S. Shortwave Diathermy. In Kitchen S. and Bazin S. eds, Clayton's Electrotherapy 10th edition, London, WB Saunders Company Ltd 1996:154-178.

Selkowitz D.M. High frequency electrical stimulation in muscle strengthening, Am J Sports Med 1989;17:103-10.

Stephenson R., Johnson M. The analgesic effects of interferential therapy on cold-induced pain in healthy subjects: A preliminary report. Physiotherapy Theory and Practice 1995;11:89-95.

Travell J.G., Simons D.G. Myofascial Pain and Dysfunction-The Trigger Point Manual. Baltimore, Williams & Wilkins 1983.

Walsh D.M. TENS: Clinical Applications and Related Theory. Singapore, Churchill Livingstone 1997.

Watson T. Electrical stimulation for wound healing. In Kitchen S. and Bazin S. eds, Clayton's Electrotherapy 10th edition, London, WB Saunders Company Ltd 1996:323-48.

Young S. Ultra-sound Therapy. In Kitchen S. and Bazin S. eds, Clayton's Electrotherapy 10th edition, London, WB Saunders Company Ltd, 1996:243-67.

Suggested reading list:

Belanger A.Y. Neuromuscular electrostimulation in physiotherapy: a critical appraisal of controversial issues. Physiotherapy Theory and Practice 1991;7:83-9.

Hobbs B. The application of electricity to acupuncture needles: a review of the current literature and research with a brief outline of the principles involved, Contemporary Therapies in Medicine 1994;2:36-40.

Holmes M.A.M., Rudland J.R. Clinical trials of ultra-sound treatment in soft tissue injury: a review and critique. Physiotherapy Theory and Practice 1991;7:163-75.

Kitchen S., Partridge C. Review of shortwave diathermy continuous and pulsed patterns. Physiotherapy 1992;78:243-52.

Marchand S., Charest J., Li J., Chenard J., Lavignolle B., Laurencelle L. Is TENS purely a placebo effect? A controlled study on chronic low back pain. Pain 1993;54:99-106.

Snyder-Mackler L., Robinson A.J. Clinical Electrophysiology: Electrotherapy and Electrophysiologic Testing. Baltimore: Williams & Wilkins 1989.

Baldry P.E. Acupuncture, Trigger Points and Musculoskeletal Pain. Edinburgh, London, Madrid, Churchill Livingstone 1993.

Janda V. Muscles and cervicogenic pain syndromes. In Grant R. ed, Physical Therapy of The Cervical and Thoracic Spine. New York: Churchill Livingston 1988: 153-66.

CHAPTER 14

EXERCISE THERAPY FOR CERVICAL SPINAL DISORDERS

Herman M.C. Lau

INTRODUCTION

Traditionally, patients with cervical spinal disorders have been treated with cervical collars, cervical traction, ultrasound, electric stimulation and manual therapy (Basmajian, 1984; Gustavsen, 1985; Maitland, 1991). These treatment modalities may form an integral part of the treatment at the early stage, but they rely on the therapist rather than the active participation of patients. Moreover, many treatment prescribed by chiropractors, doctors and physiotherapists are aimed at alleviating symptoms and are seldom aimed at preventing the recurrence of problems (McKenzie, 1995).

Rehabilitation of patients with cervical spinal disorders requires a comprehensive and holistic approach. The rehabilitation programme should involve the patient's active participation in order to be successful. Exercise therapy has an important role to play in the management of cervical spinal disorders and may be used to:

(a) restore the strength of muscles which is weakened due to disuse, for example around an inflamed joint or after injury,
(b) restore joint mobility/increase the range of movement after muscle injury,
(c) correct postural faults,
(d) prevent joint deformity and
(e) improve joint stability.

The major purpose of exercise therapy is to restore function in the treatment of musculoskeletal disorders (Corrigan & Maitland, 1983). Many therapists may underestimate the importance of exercise therapy in the treatment of cervical spinal disorders. Therefore, the aim of this chapter is to introduce the basic concepts and principles of practice of cervical exercise, which can be an effective means to treat patients with cervical spinal disorders.

EXERCISE THERAPY

Exercise therapy is the use of patient's body movement to achieve specific therapeutic effects. A clinical reasoning approach is the key to optimise the planning and execution of a successful treatment programme. To be effective, an exercise programme requires:

I.   assessment
II. individualisation
III. motivation
IV. supervision
V. evaluation and modification.

Assessment

Prior to the commencement of an exercise programme, an accurate and thorough assessment of patient's physical and functional capacity must be taken. Assessment should include the following items:

(a) History ~ general information about the musculoskeletal disorders.
(b) Observation ~ posture in sitting, standing and if possible at work.
(c) Palpation ~ palpate the soft tissue of the neck to look for any muscle spasm, atrophy or hypertrophy and assess the passive accessory intervertebral movement.
(d) Active and passive range of motion of cervical spine and related joints.
(e) Isometric muscle testing ~ neck flexion, extension, side-flexion and rotation. Pain or weakness must be noted
(f) Radiological assessment results.
(g) Functional capacity evaluation ~ assessment should pinpoint to the patient's needs, physical capacity and work requirement.

    The extent of the physical examination depends on the severity, irritability and stability of the condition. The information obtained from the assessment will form the basis of exercise programme planning.

Individualisation

Whenever an exercise programme is planned, therapists should consider the patient as a whole and should not simply consider a clinical condition affecting the cervical spine and the upper limbs only. Each exercise programme must be designed to accommodate individual needs, lifestyle, the nature of work and available training time. Therapists should monitor the progress of patients and make modifications in treatment whenever necessary. Home exercises should be simple and can be performed with a minimal amount of equipment.

Motivation

A detailed explanation of the therapy aims is required. The exercise programme must be interactive. Therapists should get the patient's participation at every stage of his treatment. His expectations and main problems should be identified. Any unrealistic expectations of the patient must be discussed and explained to patients so that they will not be disappointed and lose their motivation.

Supervision

Therapists should monitor the patient's process regularly to ensure that the prescribed exercises are properly carried out. They should correct and encourage the patient when necessary.

Evaluation and modification

The patients' progression should be regularly reviewed so that modification of exercises can be made whenever necessary. A good cervical exercise programme should produce the desired outcomes without causing fatigue or prolonged aching.

POSTURAL RE-EDUCATION

Good postural habits are important to avoid recurrence of cervical problems. In the lateral view of the neck, there is a small inward curve in the neck just above the shoulder girdle (Figure 1a), which is known as cervical lordosis. When sitting upright, the head should be directly above the shoulder girdle with a gentle cervical lordosis. Poor posture and dysfunctional movement patterns will alter the normal functions of cervical vertebrae, which may cause abnormal thoracic kyphosis and round shoulders (Sweeney, 1992). The common features of people with poor posture include head hanging in front of their body with their chin poking forward and rounded shoulders (Figure 1b).

Postural Stress

When stress due to poor posture is applied to normal tissue, it can cause pain without tissue damage. However, this can be reduced or prevented by postural re-education and relaxation exercises. As postural pain is caused by prolonged static loading upon body tissues, the pain will gradually subside when the causes of stress have been stopped This often occurs by a mere change of position (McKenzie, 1990). Prolonged neck flexion will stretch the posterior structures and compress the anterior structures of the cervical spine. If abnormal postural stresses are not relieved, patients may sometimes complain of pain either in their neck or arms despite the application of intensive treatment.

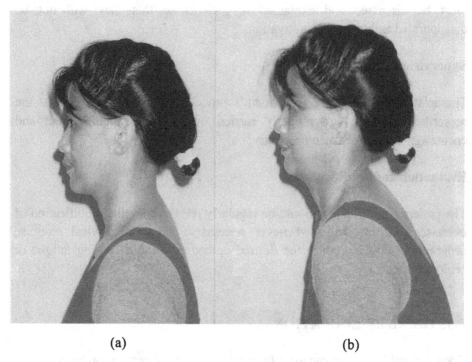

(a)   (b)

Figure 1. Comparison of different neck postures: (a) good neck posture showing a normal cervical lordosis, (b) bad neck posture

Balanced posture and developing self-awareness

A balanced posture is the state of muscular and skeletal balance that protects supporting structures of the body against injury or progressive deformity (Bland, 1987). In postural re-education, the first step is to gain the patient's co-operation and develop his or her self-awareness to facilitate changes. Development of self-awareness can be done by using a variety of biofeedback mechanisms. Video recording can be useful to assess the patient's posture and movement patterns. The patient and therapist can then discuss the findings together when the videotape is played back. Repeated assessment of posture with this method can also be helpful in checking the patient's progress. Electromyography (EMG) biofeedback machines is another useful tool for postural re-education and the application of biofeedback in postural re-education will be discussed in other textbooks.

In clinical practice, a mirror is probably the simplest equipment for providing visual feedback to patients. At the beginning of the training, the patient can either sit or stand in front of a mirror or with their side to it. These positions enable patients to see their own postural deviations.

Therapists can then identify the postural deviations to patients and assist them to find a neutral balanced position of the spine. Instructions can be verbal, with subtle hands-on cueing. It is important to assess postures that are relevant to the patient's problem.

The standing posture should be assessed because the position of the pelvis, lumbar spine and thoracic spine can significantly affect the alignment of the cervical spine and vice versa. Assessment of sitting posture is also important, particularly when the patient's symptoms are related to the sitting position, as in the case of a computer programmer who has neck pain.

Once posture has been carefully assessed, some assumptions can be made about the length and length-tension properties of key muscles. For example, a patient with forward head posture may have a lengthened longus cervicis because of the increased cervical lordosis created by this posture. Likewise, there may be shortening of the sternocleidomastoid, scalene, trapezius and/or levator scapulae muscles, since these muscles are all in a shortened position when there is an increased lordosis (White and Sahrmann, 1994). Specific stretching exercises should be included in the rehabilitation programme in order to prevent recurrence of the problems.

STRETCHING EXERCISE

A stretching exercise is defined as a therapeutic manoeuvre which can lengthen (elongate) pathologically shortened soft tissue structures and thereby increase the range of motion (Kisner and Colby, 1996). As an unrestricted and pain-free range of motions is required to perform many daily activities, it is important to have mobile and flexible periarticular soft tissues such as muscles, connective tissues and skin.

Good mobility of soft tissues and joints is also thought to be an important factor for preventing injury (Kisner and Colby, 1996). If patients are unable to achieve a balanced cervical posture due to soft tissue tightness or joint stiffness, mobilising and stretching exercises are therefore suggested to be included in their rehabilitation programme.

Principles of application

(a) The starting position of the patient should be comfortable and stable, e.g. sitting on a chair with back support.
(b) Use relaxation techniques prior to stretching if necessary.
(c) The stretching force must be strong enough to produce adequate tension on the soft tissue structures. Over-stretching should be avoided as this may cause pain or damage to the structures.
(d) The stretching force must be provided in a sustained manner. Ballistic stretching tends to cause the greatest amount of injury to tissues.
(e) The duration of holding the stretch should be around 15 to 30 seconds.
(f) The stretch should be released gradually.
(g) Short rest periods should be allowed.
(h) If there are any signs and symptoms of vertebral artery insufficiency, stretching exercises should be stopped

Examples of stretching exercise (Kisner and Colby, 1996)

Tight anterior chest, scapular and humeral musculature are usually found in patients with poor cervical and thoracic posture. Levator scapulae, sternocleido-mastoid, latissimus dorsi and shoulder internal rotator muscles are the key muscles to work on to the neck posture.

Therapists are therefore encouraged to apply their functional anatomy knowledge to prescribe specific stretching exercises for individual patients. Some stretching exercises commonly used in the management of cervical spinal disorders are illustrated as follows:

(a) To stretch the side flexors of the neck

Sitting on a firm and straight backed chair, the patient is asked to perform axial extension (tuck the chin in and straighten the neck) and then bend the neck to the opposite side from tight muscles. To stretch the neck, patient can use the hand of the opposite side to apply a stretching force over the temporal area of the head (Figure 2a).

(b) To stretch the neck rotators

Using the same starting position as in (a), the patient is asked to perform axial extension (tuck the chin in and straighten the neck) and then turn his head to the side where movement is limited. Stretching force can be applied with one hand on the cheek and the other hand on the back of the head. (Figure 2b). The patient will feel the stretching on the side of the neck.

(c) To stretch the neck extensors

Using the same starting position as in (a) again, the patient is asked to clasp his hands at the back of the upper neck and perform axial extension (tucking the chin in and straightening the neck) and then bring his chin down to the chest. Stretching force can be applied through the hands to the neck (Figure 2c). Stretch will be felt in the lower neck and the upper back.

(d) To stretch the neck flexors

The patient is asked to sit on a firm and high backed chair to perform axial extension (tuck the chin in and straighten the neck) and then tilt his head backwards. Patient should put a finger on his chin as a reminder to retain the retraction while moving into extension. Stretching force can be applied with a hand over the forehead (Figure 2d).

(e) To stretch the upper trapezius

The patient is asked to sit on a firm and straight backed chair in front of a mirror. Then, he can perform axial extension (tuck the chin in and straighten the neck), bend of the neck to the opposite side of the tight upper trapezius muscle with the head turned to the same side and bend forward. For example, to stretch the right upper trapezius, the patient has to laterally flex to the left, rotate to the right and flex forward. Gentle stretching force may be applied with the palm of the left hand placed over the right temporo-occipital area of the head.

(f) To stretch the scalene muscles

The patient is asked to stand next to a table and hold on its edge. While doing axial extension (tuck the chin in and straighten the neck), the patient bends his neck to the opposite side of the tight muscles and rotates towards the same side. To stretch the muscle, the patient leans away from the table, inhales, exhales and holds the stretch position.

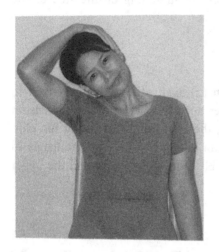

Figure 2a. Lateral flexion to the right with overpressure.

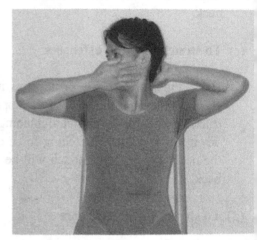

Figure 2b. Rotation to the right with overpressure.

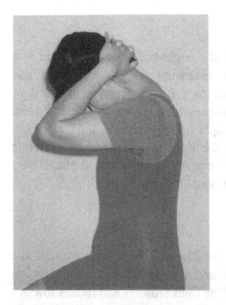

Figure 2c. Forward flexion with overpressure to stretch the extensors.

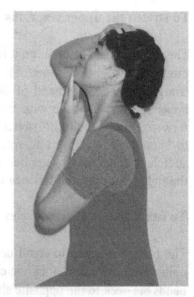

Figure 2d. Extension performed in the retracted position.

(g) To stretch the suboccipital muscles

With the same starting position as in (a), patients are asked to use the thumb of the dominant hand to stabilise the spinous process of the second cervical vertebra. To stretch the muscle, the patient is asked to nod his head slowly to perform a tipping motion of the head upon the upper cervical spine.

(h) To stretch the anterior chest muscles

The patient is asked to lie on his back with hands behind the head and elbows resting on the mattress. To increase the stretch, a small firm pillow can be placed under the thoracic spine between the scapulae. To combine the stretch exercise with breathing, the patient can take a breath in while bringing his elbows down to the mattress and holding this posture for a few seconds. Elbows can then be relaxed and brought together when breathing out.

STRENGTHENING EXERCISE

A strengthening exercise is a kind of resisted active exercise, which involves either dynamic or static muscular contraction against a manual or mechanical resistance. Muscle strengthening exercises can either be isometric, isotonic or isokinetic.

Isometric exercise does not involve joint motion and therefore this is indicated for patients with painful or unstable cervical spines. Isotonic exercise involves joint motion against resistance. Isokinetic exercise also involves resisted joint motion, but the speed of motion is fixed during exercise. However, special isokinetic equipment (e.g. Cybex) is required.

Multifidi are important interspinal muscles for maintaining the normal functions of the cervical spine. Therefore, multifidi strengthening exercises should not be ignored, particularly in preventing the recurrence of cervical spinal problems. As multifidi are small muscles, exercise intensity should be light and exercise instruction should be detailed enough to avoid training the sternocleidomastoid or anterior neck muscles (Hertling and Kessler, 1996). If the exercise resistance is more than 40% of the maximum voluntary contraction of the muscle, inappropriate synergistic muscles are likely to be involved (Richardson, 1992).

Principles of application

(a) The patient should be positioned in a stable and comfortable position.
(b) The neck and upper extremities should be free from restrictive clothing.
(c) In order to optimise the strengthening effect, exercise should not cause pain.
(d) Movements should be smooth when doing dynamic resisted exercise.
(e) Resistance should be applied and released gradually.

Examples of strengthening exercise

(a) Cervical isometric exercises

In this exercise, the patient is required to stand next to a wall. Using a book, he will be asked to keep the neck in a neutral position while firm pressure is applied to strengthen the neck muscles isometrically (Figures 3a, 3b, 3c).

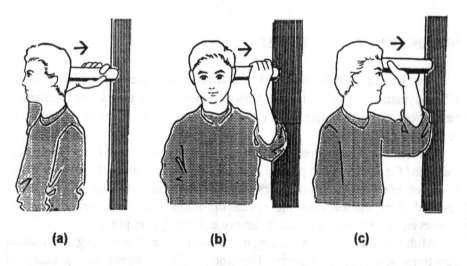

(a)   **(b)**   **(c)**

Figure 3. Isometric strengthening of (a) neck extensors, (b) neck side flexors & (c) neck flexors.

(b) Isometric strengthening of the multifidus muscle

The patients is required to sit on a firm and comfortable straight backed chair. A hand is then cupped behind the neck, forming a slight backward curve. Light pressure is applied to the back of the head and the patient is asked to hold this position for a while (Figure 4a).

(c) Specific segmental strengthening exercise of multifidus muscle

Using the same starting position in (b), patient will be asked to place two fingers at the level to be strengthened and then bring his neck backwards and sideways over the fingers. The patient is asked to hold this position while force is applied to the opposite side. For progression, this exercise can be repeated with around 10 degrees of motion allowance (Figure 4b).

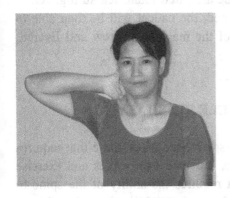 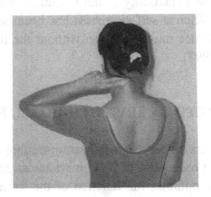

Figure 4a. Isometric strengthening of multifidus.

Figure 4b. Specific segmental strengthening of multifidus.

RELAXATION EXERCISE

When muscle contracts too suddenly, tension will build up in the golgi tendon organs of the muscle. This will stimulate an inverse stretch reflex. Impulses from the golgi tendon organs will then pass to the spinal cord and synapse through alpha motor neurones to fire the muscle with inhibitory impulses. If the force of the contraction is strong, these impulses will inhibit muscle contraction and lead to a period of relaxation (Fox, 1996).

If prolonged flexion is required by patients' jobs, this posture will increase the muscle tension in the upper trapezius or neck extensor muscles. In order to treat these patients, the first step is to ask the patient to shrug his shoulders upwards and then contract his upper trapezius maximally. A period of relaxation will then follow which should be at least as long as the contraction time. Patient should be asked to learn the relaxation sensation so as to reproduce it on his own.

Suggested verbal commands:
(a) Shrug your shoulders upwards.
(b) Tighten the muscle.
(c) Breathe in deeply and then hold it.
(d) Exhale slowly from your mouth and relax the shoulders as much as you can.

EMG biofeedback can be used in conjunction with this method. It will give specific information about the tension of individual muscle groups. This will help patients to control their muscles with confidence. Instant feedback and impartiality of the machine's response are often found reassuring. Once sufficient self-awareness has been developed, the patient will be then able to reduce muscle tension without the help of the machine. (Trew and Everett, 1997).

ACTIVE CERVICOTHORACIC MUSCLE STABILISATION

Cervicothoracic stabilisation training is a specialised programme that requires co-ordination of body mechanics, posture, movement principles and exercise to optimise the function of the spine. It requires the ability of the spine to restore its neutral position and the appropriate use of stabilisation principles.

Stabilisation training optimises the capacity of the cervicothoracic spine to absorb loads in all directions. Therefore, it can minimise direct stress and strain on individual cervical tissues (Sweeney, 1992). Initial training of active cervicothoracic stabilisation exercises include a series of isolated exercises in the cervical, interscapular, chest and upper extremity musculature. As the patient progresses, exercise within the tolerance of neck pain can be done. Some suggested exercises are explained below. However, modifications should be made to meet the individual patient's need.

(a) To strengthen the axial extensor and thoracic extensor, the patient will be asked to tuck his chin in while standing with hips and knees bent. As he moves his arms, the patient is required to stabilise the head and neck actively (Figure 5).

(b) To strengthen the cervical flexors, the patient will be asked to stand up and use his forehead to hold an inflatable ball, about the size of a basketball, against the wall. As he moves his arms, the patient is asked to actively stabilise the neck and head (Figure 6).

(c) In order to train the cervical muscles, the patient is asked to stand up and uses his forehead to hold the inflatable ball against the wall again. Then, the patient is then asked to roll the ball along the wall with his head. This exercise requires the patient to turn his body as he walks along.

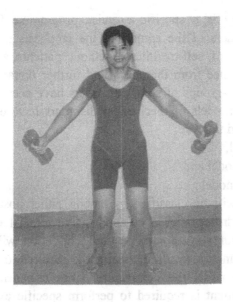

Figure 5. Active stabilisation exercise for cervical and thoracic extensors.

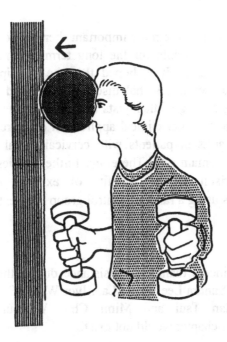

Figure 6. Active stabilisation exercise for cervical flexors.

MCKENZIE THERAPY FOR CERVICAL SPINAL DISORDERS

McKenzie therapy is a specific exercise programme for the treatment of mechanical disorders of the spine and the emphasis is self treatment. By teaching a series of self-treatment method, patients are then expected to achieve independence from therapists and further therapy (McKenzie 1990). Three specific sub-groups of spinal disorders have been identified Therefore, three conceptual models of mechanical disorders have been proposed in the therapy course and they are:

(1) postural model,
(2) dysfunction model and
(3) derangement model.

The patient will be classified as having either postural, dysfunction or derangement syndrome after a comprehensive clinical examination. For a patient with postural syndrome, postural correction will be given. For a patient with dysfunction syndrome, patient is required to do specific exercises to stretch and remodel the contracture. For a patient with derangement syndrome, the patient is required to perform specific exercises to reduce or centralise the displacement.

SUMMARY

Exercise therapy is one of the most important therapeutic methods in physical medicine and is indispensable for the long term treatment of patients with cervical spinal disorders. It is hoped that the principles and practice of exercise therapy for cervical spinal disorders discussed in this chapter will improve the understanding of therapists and provide them with guidelines to follow. Despite the fact that clinical application of exercise therapy provides good long term results in patients with cervical spinal disorders, scientific studies in this area remain rare. Therefore, further studies are encouraged. In particular, comparison of the benefits of exercise therapy with other therapeutical agents using a random control group is essential.

Acknowledgements

My grateful and sincere thanks for assistance during the production of this chapter must go to Sandra Lee, Jamie Lau, Ivor Wong, Edwin Lee, April Lam, Aaron Smith, Alan Tsui and Mimi Chu. Without their advice and encouragement, this chapter would not exist.

References:

Basmajian J.V. Therapeutic Exercise. Baltimore, Williams and Wilkins 1984.

Bland J.H. Disorders of the Cervical Spine. Philadelphia, W.B. Saunders, 1987.

Corrigan B. and Maitland G.D. Practical Orthopaedic Medicine. London, Butterworth 1983.

Fox S.I. Human Physiology, Fifth edition, Boston, WC Brown 1996.

Gustavsen R. Training Therapy: Prophylaxis and Rehabilitation. New York, Thieme, 1985.

Hertling D. and Kessler R.M. Management of Common Musculo-skeletal Disorders. Third edition, Philadelphia, Lippincott 1996.

Kisner C., Colby L.A. Therapeutic Exercise, Third edtion, Philadelphia, F.A. Davis Company 1996.

Maitland G.D. Vertebral Manipulation. Third edition, London, Butterworths 1991.

McKenzie R. The Cervical and Thoracic Spine. New Zealand, Spinal Publications (NZ) Ltd. 1990.

McKenzie R. Treat Your Own Neck. Second edition, New Zealand, Spinal Publications 1995.

Richardson C. Muscle Imbalance: Principles of Treatment and Assessment. Proceedings of the New Zealand Society of Physiotherapists Challenges Conference, Churchill, August 1992.

Sweeney T. Neck School: Cervicothoracic Stabilisation Training Occupational Medicine 1992,7:43-54.

Trew M. and Everett T. Human Movement. Third edition, Churchill Livingstone, New York, 1997.

White S.G. and Sahrmann S.A. In: Grant ER ed, Physical Therapy of the Cervical and Thoracic Spine. New York, Churchill Livingstone 1994.

Suggested reading list:

Barton P.M., Hayes K.C. Neck Flexor Muscle Strength, Efficiency and Relaxation Times in Normal Subjects and Subjects with Unilateral Neck Pain and Headache. Arch Phys Med Rehabil 1996;27:680-7.

Calliet R. Neck and Arm Pain. Third editon, Philadelphia, FA Davis 1991.

Donatelli R.A., Wooden M.J. Orthopaedic Physical Therapy. Second edition, New York, Churchill Livingstone 1994.

Grant R. Physical Therapy of the Cervical and Thoracic Spine. Second edition, Churchill, Livingstone, 1994.

Highland T.R., Dreisinger T.E., Vie L.L., Russell G.S. Changes in Isometric
        Strength and Range of Motion of the Isolated Cervical Spine After
        Eight Weeks of Clinical Rehabilitation. Spine 1992;17:77-82.
Pollock M.L.   Frequency and Volume of Resistance Training: Effect on
        Cervical Extension Strength. Arch Phys Med Rehabil 1993;74:1080-6.

CHAPTER 15

MANUAL THERAPY FOR CERVICAL SPINAL DISORDERS

Ella W. Yeung

MANUAL THERAPY FOR CERVICAL SPINAL DISORDERS

This chapter discusses the basic principles of the use of manual therapy in the assessment and management of cervical spine disorders. Manual therapy refers to the process of examination and the application of manual (passive mobilisation or manipulation) techniques. Passive mobilisation utilises low velocity pressure performed within or at the limit of joint range of movement (Grieve, 1994). Manipulation involves a sudden forceful movement or high velocity thrust to a specific joint level (Maitland, 1986).

EXAMINATION OF THE CERVICAL SPINE

The assessment procedure forms an essential part of manual therapy. It has always been the keystone in developing working hypotheses and in critical analysis of a patient's problem. Maitland (1986) has contributed significantly in devising a systematic and logical method for clinical examination. The approach emphasises that examination, techniques and assessment are interrelated.

CLINICAL REASONING PROCESS

In order to make sense of the information provided by the patient, a sound clinical reasoning process is required. Jones (1992) has provided a very useful framework of the clinical reasoning process for physiotherapists. The model proposed relies on hypothetico-deductive reasoning which involve hypothesis generation, testing and modification. Three core elements have been identified

(Jones, 1997) to be essential for effective clinical reasoning: the use of knowledge, the act of cognition and the process of metacognition (i.e. awareness and monitoring of cognition). The process begins from the encounter with patient, the way he enters the room, the way he speaks, information from the referral notes, combined with successive detection of both verbal and non-verbal cues. This process leads to a small array of initial hypotheses and possibly goes on from this to actual solutions of the clinical problem. As working hypotheses develop, they are then tested by further relevant questions and by specific tests unique to patient's presentation. Jones (1992) has suggested the use of five hypothesis categories as a strategy to guide the reasoning process. They are (1) source(s) of symptoms or dysfunction; (2) contributing factors; (3) precautions and contra-indications to physical examination and treatment; (4) management; and (5) prognosis. The examination procedure consists of patient inquiry/interview and physical examination. The patient inquiry involves the patient's account of his complaint and the physical examination encompasses the use of different test procedures.

PATIENT INTERVIEW

The information obtained from the interview will help physiotherapists to establish the kind of disorders, the severity and irritability of disorders and precautions/cautions required to take during physical examination (Magarey, 1994).

Main complaint

The patient's main problem or complaint should be first identified, followed by a detailed recording of the symptoms on a body chart. Detailed descriptions of the site, depth, severity, the quality and frequency of the symptoms should be sought from the patient. This information is useful to identify the source of symptoms. Superficial somatic, deep somatic, neurogenic, viscerogenic referred and psychogenic pain have their own characteristics and qualities. Since the patient's complaint is a symptom and not a diagnosis, the identification of the sources or pathological process depends on the physiotherapist's knowledge and clinical interpretation ability. The source of neck pain is beyond the scope of discussion in this chapter; useful references are available for readers who would like to increase their understanding in this area (Aprill *et al.*, 1990; Dwyer *et al.*, 1990; Grant, 1994; Grieve, 1994; Borenstein *et al.*, 1996).

Behaviour of symptoms

Assessment of symptoms behaviour should include questions on the aggravating, alleviating factors, relationship between symptoms and their 24-hour patterns. Mechanical causes of cervical pain are frequently associated with a specific activity performed in a mechanically disadvantaged position (Borenstein *et al.*, 1996). It usually worsens with an increase in that activity and eases with rest. Careful analysis of the particular movement, activity or position together with knowledge of functional anatomy will enable the physiotherapist to build up a clinical picture of the patient and form working hypotheses. To determine the severity of the patient's disorder, three aspects of the behaviour of patient's symptoms related to a particular function or activity need to be sought (Maitland, 1986). Physiotherapists should determine (1) the activity that provokes the symptoms, (2) the severity of symptoms caused by the activity and (3) the duration for symptoms to subside. This information will then determine which kind of physical examination should be carried out. If the disorder is irritable, physical examination techniques will be limited in order to prevent exacerbation of symptoms. The 24-hour pattern of symptoms provides useful information about the symptoms in relation to activity and rest. Patients with inflammatory arthropathies usually complain of morning stiffness which eases with movement (Borenstein *et al.*, 1996). Physiotherapists should be cautious of the possibility of a more sinister disorder if symptoms are constant and unrelieved/worsened by rest (Magarey, 1994).

Precautionary questions

Questions regarding to the patient's general health, relevant weight loss, radiographs and medications should be posed so as to ascertain any precautions or contra-indications to physical examination and treatment. For the cervical spine, information about the presence/absence of dizziness and spinal cord symptoms should also be obtained from the patient (Maitland, 1986).

History of the complaint

A thorough review of patient's history is essential to understanding the patient's problem. Maitland (1986) has divided history taking into four main areas: (1) the onset and development of the present episode, (2) the present stage of disorders, (3) the present stability of the disorders and (4) the previous history, including episodic development. If the history of symptoms originates from trauma, the physiotherapist should identify the mechanism of the injury in detail. If the onset of symptoms is spontaneous, the presence of any possible predisposing factors needs to be identified. If the patient had previously suffered from the same complaint, the physiotherapist should detail the first episode and successive complaints. Any information related to the patient's past treatment and its effects will assist the physiotherapist to formulate management hypotheses.

PHYSICAL EXAMINATION

The patient interview forms the initial part of symptoms evaluation. By listening to the patient's description of his complaints carefully, physiotherapist should be then able to formulate some working hypotheses. It is important to emphasise that physical examination is not a series of routine tests, but is a continuation of testing of the initial working hypotheses. Therefore, planning is necessary to determine the extent to which the examination should be performed and what types of appropriate tests are required. A musculoskeletal dysfunction is usually associated with physical impairment of the articular, neuromuscular and nervous system (Jull, 1997). Therefore, using appropriate tests, the physical examination should aim at reproducing similar symptoms, in order to determine the potential sources of symptom(s) and to identify contributing factors to the complaint (Magarey, 1994).

Observation

The resting posture of the cervical and thoracic spine should be observed from the front, from behind and at the sides of the patient. Several factors have been postulated as affecting the curvature of the cervical spine, such as thoracic kyphosis, elevation and protraction of shoulders, cervical disc narrowing, muscle spasm or derangement of the zygapophyseal joints (Gay, 1993). The amount of cervical lordosis is both age and gender dependent and there is considerable variability in cervical posture (Gore, 1986; Grimmer, 1997). Research that links a forward leaning posture of the head as the cause of abnormal load to cervical structures leading to pain are mostly anecdotal (Ayub *et al.*, 1984; Tan and Nordin, 1992). The causal relationship between poor head posture and pain has yet to be established.

Active movements

The standard movements of the cervical spine include flexion, extension, lateral flexion and rotation. Physiotherapists should establish the patient's resting symptoms before assessing the effects of these movements. During the assessment of individual movement, details of the range of movement, quality of movement, onset and location of symptoms and their relationship with symptoms should be taken into consideration. The relationship between symptoms and movement may provide important clues to physiotherapists to identify the potential source(s) of symptoms and their contributing factor(s), as well as an appropriate management plan (Jones and Jones, 1994). Overpressure is then applied for those movements that have full and pain free range. The application of overpressure helps to ensure that the movement has gone through its "true" physiological range (Grieve, 1994).

Additional test movements

If active standard movements cannot reproduce similar symptoms, varying the movements under different loading modes may be indicated. For example, one could change the speed of movements, repeat movements, sustain the movement or perform the movements under distraction/compression. It will be most valuable to analyse the symptoms provoking functional activities prompted by patient during the interview and to examine the activity in either isolation or with different combinations of movement. In addition, each component of that combined movement can be selectively loaded to define the cause of dysfunction (Edwards, 1992; Grieve, 1994; Magarey, 1994).

Passive physiologic intervertebral movement (PPIVMs) tests

The range and quality of movement of individual spinal segments can be examined using PPIVMs. The purpose of the tests is to detect any restriction of physiological movement at each vertebral level, whereas motion disorders may be not obvious on gross movement tests (Magarey, 1994). Detailed descriptions of these tests can be found in other texts [e.g. Grieve (1994) and Maitland (1994)].

Neurological examination

The cervical neurological examination consists of three aspects: motor strength testing, reflex examination and sensation testing. Any compression or traction of nerve root will cause motor weakness, decrease of reflex function and change/decrease in various degrees of sensation. It has been suggested that true muscle weakness is one of the most reliable indicators of persistent nerve compression, whereas sensory changes may be rather subjective and reflexes can be difficult to test with increasing age (Borenstein *et al.*, 1996). Motor strength examination can be helpful in assessing muscles innervated by different nerve roots of the cervical spine. The deltoid is innervated by C5 and biceps strength determines the integrity of the C6 nerve root. The C7 level is tested by evaluating the triceps, whereas C8 innervation can be evaluated by testing the long finger flexors and extensor pollicis longus. The intrinsic muscles can be tested to determine the T1 neurological level. The biceps reflex primarily tests the integrity of the C5 nerve root and the triceps reflex predominately tests the C7 nerve root. Sensation testing involves the examination of light touch sensation. If abnormalities are found, sensation tests can be done. Areas with decreased/altered sensation should be recorded for future reassessment.

Neurodynamic tests

As the nervous system is a continuum, this is fundamental to understand the use of neurodynamic tests. Butler (1991) highlighted that the nervous system will adapt to tension produced by movement and stretch. In the event of a pathological process, this may lead to abnormal tension and cause symptoms. The neural component of patient's disorder can therefore be identified by neurodynamic-based tests, such as the slump test and upper limb tension test. These tests are discussed in detail by Butler (1991).

Palpation

Palpation of the cervical spine is an important aspect of the examination. In performing palpation assessment, the physiotherapist should identify any thickening, swelling, muscle spasm or tightness of the soft tissues. Any bony anomalies in terms of asymmetry, deviation or prominence should be noted (Magarey, 1994). Passive accessory intervertebral movements (PAIVMs) are then examined to detect any restriction of movement, soft tissue resistance, reproduction of symptoms and to assess the quality of movement, particularly at the end range of motion. The direction of PAVIM can be varied, but the most commonly employed procedures are posteroanterior and anteroposterior oscillatory pressure applied when the patient is in prone and supine positions respectively. There have been concerns raised regarding the validity of palpation. It seems that experienced physiotherapists are usually able to discriminate and make correct judgements. In a study that compared manual examination of cervical zygapophyseal joint findings with radiographic assessment (Jull *et al.*, 1988), the physiotherapist identified accurately all the 15 patients who had symptomatic joint involvement and the other five who did not have joint involvement. However, in another study performed by Maher and Adams (1995), the investigators attempted to evaluate the physiotherapists' ability to assess stiffness. Their results showed a poor to fair reliability. It was suggested that the concept of stiffness is multidimensional and the individual's concept of stiffness is different. Hence, physiotherapists need to improve the operational definitions of stiffness (Mahar, 1995; Mahar and Adams, 1995).

Muscle testing

It has been postulated that forward head posture is associated with tightness in the deep neck extensors, scaleni, levator scapulae, trapezius, sternocleido-mastoid, pectoral and shoulder medial rotators muscles and weakness of the deep cervical flexors, long cervical extensors, lower scapular stabilisers and shoulder lateral rotators (Magarey, 1994). If the results of the patient interview suggest that muscles may be a potential source of symptoms, the physiotherapist should examine these structures.

Vertebro-basilar artery insufficiency (VBI) test

Patients who present a history of dizziness or other associated symptoms, such as drop attacks, diplopia, dysarthria, dysphagia, nauseous and vomiting, should be appropriately tested for vertebral artery insufficiency (Grant, 1994). Details of the procedures on pre-manipulative testing of the cervical spine are outlined in the Australian Physiotherapy Association protocol in 1988. If any of the tests can reproduce dizziness or other associated symptoms, then cervical manipulation should not be done.

Examination of associated structures

Other joints or associated structures which may contribute to the patient's symptoms should be assessed. Examples of these are the thoracic spine and the scapulohumeral complex. Other examination procedures such as cervical quadrant tests, thoracic outlet tests, palpation of the first rib may be necessary if these structures are implicated as potential source(s) of symptoms.

ASSESSMENT AND TREATMENT PRINCIPLES

As discussed earlier, assessment of the patient's problem is an ongoing process throughout the whole examination. Assessment should be continued during the application and at the conclusion of treatment. In addition, a good understanding of the biomechanics, functional anatomy, pain patterns and pathological process is also essential. Treatment strategy is formulated after the analysis of the information and after the working hypotheses have been re-defined and re-ranked.

It is important to understand that deciding on the treatment is directed towards determining clinical problems within the scope of physiotherapy. It is based on clinical criteria, such as limitation of accessory range of movement, soft tissue abnormalities, instead of treating the 'pathology'. This is because similar clinical diagnoses can have different clinical findings (Maitland, 1986). Particular attention should be paid to the pain response patterns during movements testing as this can assist in the selection of passive movement techniques (Trott, 1994).

The grades of passive mobilisation are defined by Maitland (1986) as follows: Grade I is mobilisation performed at the beginning of the joint range with a small amplitude movement; Grade II is mobilisation performed with a large amplitude movement in a resistance free part of the range; a large amplitude movement performed to the point of approximately 50% of resistance is defined as Grade III, whereas a small amplitude movement performed to the point of approximately 50% of resistance is defined as Grade IV. Grade V movement refers to a high velocity thrust performed at the limit of the joint range of movement.

If pain is the only factor limiting movement, the use of either accessory or physiological movements (e.g. Grade I and II) without provoking symptoms is recommended. For a patient showing only tissue resistance as the factor limiting movement, passive mobilisation techniques (either physiological or accessory) in the most severely restricted direction or manipulation can be considered. When both pain and resistance are present during movement, the grades of mobilisation will depend upon the severity, quality and behaviour of pain associated with the resistance (Jones *et al.*, 1994). The selection of grades, direction, frequency and duration of passive mobilisation will depend on the hypotheses made about the need for caution in the patient interview, the relationship between quality of movement and the symptoms produced during the application of particular passive movement (Jones *et al.*, 1994).

Manual treatment techniques via the nervous system mobilisation (i.e. neurodynamic tests) can also be utilised if there are clues showing that the mechanics of the nervous system are altered or the possible structures around and along the nervous system have interfered with normal mechanics (Butler, 1991). For further discussion of these concepts, readers can refer to Maitland (1986), Butler (1991), Jones *et al.* (1994) and Trott (1994).

TREATMENT MODALITIES

The most common treatment modalities for cervical spinal disorders are mobilisation, manipulation and cervical traction in manual therapy. Attempts have been made to examine the implication of use of these modalities and their efficacy. Mobilisation of the neural tissues via neurodynamic tests is also a useful treatment tool. However readers need to understand the underlying rationale of this treatment in order to make it clinically applicable. This concept is discussed in great detail by Butler (1991).

There are several conditions of which manipulation is contra-indicated. They include osteoporosis, osteomyelitis, malignancy, recent fractures, cord and cauda equina syndromes, inflammatory arthopathy (e.g. rheumatoid arthritis, ankylosing spondylitis), vertebro-basilar artery insufficiency, spondylolisthesis and gross foraminal encroachment. The last four conditions listed above are not absolutely contra-indicated to mobilisation and cervical traction, but extreme care must be taken to avoid exacerbation (Maitland, 1986).

MOBILISATION / MANIPULATION

Spinal mobilisation and manipulation are widely used for the treatment of cervical dysfunction. On examination of the clinical efficacy of manual techniques, Ottenbacher and Di Fabio (1985) conducted a meta-analysis while Koes *et al.* (1991) presented a critical review of 35 randomised clinical trials to compare spinal manipulation with other treatments. Both studies concluded that there is only limited empirical support in this area and the effectiveness of manipulation techniques are controversial. Two studies (Cassidy *et al.*, 1992; Koes *et al.*, 1992) are presented below for readers' interest. It has been suggested that further research with a better methodological design and which focus on the long term effects in patients with more specific conditions are needed (Koes *et al.*; 1991;1992). The immediate effect of manipulation versus mobilisation in neck pain patients was compared using a randomised controlled trial (Cassidy *et al.*, 1992). Subjects who suffered from mechanical neck pain with radial pain spreading down to the trapezius muscles were selected for the study. Their results showed that both types of treatment increased the range of movement. However, manipulation achieved a greater effect on pain relief than mobilisation. Koes *et al.* (1992) performed a randomised clinical trial in patients with chronic neck and back pain, to compare the effectiveness of manual therapy (mobilisation and manipulation), conventional physiotherapy (exercises, massage and electrical modalities), treatment received by general practitioners alone (medication, advice) and placebo treatment (detuned shortwave diathermy and detuned ultrasound). At 12 months' follow up, results indicated that manual therapy group had the largest improvement in terms of change in the patient's main complaints. Furthermore, physical functioning seemed to improve consistently with the manual therapy group, although the level of changes was not statistically significant. Another extra finding was that the number of treatment was considerably less in the manual therapy group as compared with the conventional physiotherapy group. Subgroup analysis suggested that great improvement is common in chronic patients with a history of exhibiting the complaint for more than one year and in patients who were younger than 40 (Koes *et al.*, 1993).

Proposed effects of manual therapy

It has been proposed by Wyke (1985) that spinal manual therapy influences the mechanoreceptive input which then subsequently leads to a decrease in muscle tension. It is proposed that activation of spinal interneurones as a result of peripheral mechanoreceptor stimulation, such as joint or soft tissue manipulation, will produce presynaptic inhibition of nociceptive afferent activity. Zusman *et al.* (1994), in their studies of the effect of pain relief using combined passive movement techniques, demonstrated with chronic neck pain patients and observed that the pain threshold levels were increased after manipulation. There were other clinical studies which showed that spinal mobilisation procedures influence the sympathetic nervous system function (Peterson *et al.*, 1993; Slater *et al.*, 1994; Vicenzino *et al.*, 1994; Vernon *et al.*, 1990). Two studies by Vicenzino *et al.* (1995) and Wright and Vicenzino (1995) illustrated that mechanical pain threshold was significantly increased after two cervical mobilisation techniques. Wright (1995) in a recent article attempted to explain the analgesic effect demonstrated after spinal manipulative therapy. He proposed that the pain relieving effect might be mediated through the descending pain inhibitory system projecting from the dorsal system of the periaqueductal grey via nuclei in the ventrolateral medulla to the spinal cord. Mobilisation has been shown to improve the extensibility of connective tissue, as well as to maintain lubricating efficiency about the joint (Akeson *et al.*, 1980). Long term benefits of passive movement have been examined in numerous studies. Research findings suggested that it is effective in the restoration of range of movement, reduction of oedema, joint stiffness, capsular contractures and pain (O'Driscoll *et al.*, 1983; McCarthy *et al.*, 1992; 1993). However, there is only limited understanding of the minimum dosage of manual therapy has on the connective tissues. Threlkeld (1992) commented that the effectiveness of manipulative therapy techniques depends on the force applied, treatment duration, the region treated and the type of pathology. However, there is a paucity of literature examining these factors.

CERVICAL TRACTION

Mechanical cervical traction is another type of passive treatment modality for cervical dysfunction. It has been suggested that cervical traction is beneficial for clinical conditions, such as osteoarthritis of the vertebral joints, radicular referral, capsulitis, pathology of the anterior and posterior longitudinal ligaments and muscle spasm due to reflex mechanism (Basmajian, 1981). The proposed mechanical effects include vertebral joint separation and widening of the intervertebral foramen (Saunders, 1983; Bridger *et al.*, 1990). It has also been reported that cervical traction is helpful in improving the circulation within epidural space, loosening of adhesions within dural sleeves, reducing compression or irritation of nerve roots, separating zygapophyseal joints and reducing muscle spasm (Harris, 1977; Basmajian, 1981).

Widening of intervertebral foramen

The mode of delivery is influenced by the position of the neck, the mode of traction (constant verse intermittent), traction force, the angle of pull and the position of the patient. Several studies have attempted to look at these different variables. Colachis and Strohm (1965) studied different traction forces and suggested that the posterior vertebral separation is at its maximum (1~1.5mm per space) with traction force above 9 kg. The authors also demonstrated that the greatest spinal separation of intervertebral foramen and disc space occurred at an angle of 24° of pull with 25 to 50 lbs. of traction force. Deets *et al.* (1977) compared the effect of different starting positions in cervical traction and suggested that the supine position offers the best relaxation and less traction force is required to increase the posterior intervertebral spaces. This finding was also supported by Murphy (1991) who demonstrated that muscle activity increased in the sitting position as compared with the supine position during traction. Grieve (1994) also recommended that patient should be positioned so that the segment to be treated is at the midpoint of its available sagittal movement.

Muscle relaxation

The effects of cervical traction on muscle relaxation remain disputable. DeLarceda (1980) suggested that intermittent cervical traction (13.6 kg) is effective in producing rhythmic muscle contraction and relaxation, and hence the improvement of muscle blood flow and reduction in pain. Using sustained cervical traction mode, Klaber-Moffett *et al.* (1990b) demonstrated a reduction in myoelectric activity of upper trapezius muscle immediately after 20 minutes of traction. However, the effect was no longer significant when subjects returned to the upright position. They further showed that little or no weight seems to induce more relaxation in the muscles than applying heavy weight. Jette *et al.* (1985) compared the myoelectric activity of the upper trapezius muscle before, during and after 20 minutes of intermittent cervical traction. However, they demonstrated that cervical muscles were already relaxed in the supine position and therefore the decrease in muscle spasm migth not be an adequate explanation for the reduction of pain in cervical traction. Another study investigated (Murphy, 1991) the myoelectric activity of middle scaleni muscle during 10 minutes of intermittent cervical traction and concluded that cervical traction did not appear to produce immediate muscular relaxation.

Pain reduction

Several investigators have investigated the efficacy of cervical traction for neck pain. A study by Goldie and Landquist (1970) demonstrated that either traction or isometric exercises led to a similar degree of improvement in mobility and pain in a group of patients with cervical pain. Zylbergold and Piper (1985) performed a randomised clinical trial in 100 patients with cervical brachialgia. They demonstrated that cervical forward flexion and rotation were improved significantly in a group of patients who had received cervical traction. Intermittent traction was found to be more effective than static traction in relieving pain. In a study of 100 patients with neck and arm pain, Klaber-Moffett *et al.* (1990a) showed that patients receiving continuous traction with 6 to 15 lbs. tended to improve slightly more than a placebo group on the measures of pain, sleep disturbance, social dysfunction, activities of daily living and range of movement.

Due to differences in patient groups, treatment procedures and outcome measures, it is difficult to make a comparison between these studies. In a recent systematic analysis of the literature relating to the efficacy of traction for patients with neck or back pain (Van der Heijden *et al.*, 1995), the authors concluded that the studies currently available do not provide clear conclusions due to poor methodological designs and small sample sizes. Although there is no evidence to show that traction is ineffective, further research with proper design is needed to investigate the effect of traction.

CONCLUSIONS

This chapter has provided an overview of the use of manual therapy in cervical disorders. For physiotherapists who want to further understand the context of manual therapy, it is suggested that they can refer to the recommended references as listed below. Identification of any pathological process in the cervical spine may not necessarily correlate with the patient's symptoms. Based on careful assessment and sound clinical reasoning, manual therapy can be a very useful and effective treatment for cervical spine disorders. In order to provide patients with a holistic treatment programme and to prevent recurrence of symptoms, manual therapy must be integrated with therapeutic exercises and ergonomic advice.

References:

Akeson W.H., Amiel D., Woo S.L.Y. Immobility effects on synovial joints: the pathomechanics of joint contracture. Bioheology 1980;17:95-110.

Aprill C., Dwyer A., Bogduk N. Cervical zygapophyseal joint pain patterns II: A clinical evaluation. Spine 1990; 15:458-461.

Australian Physiotherapy Association: Protocol of pre-manipulative testing of the cervical spine. Aust J Physiotherapy 1988;34:97.

Ayub E., Glasheen-Wray M., Kraus S. Head posture: A case study of the effects of the rest position of the mandible. J Orthop Sports Phys Ther 1984;5:179-83.

Basmajian J.V. Manipulation, traction and massage. Third edition, London, Williams and Wilkins 1981.

Borenstein D.G., Wiesel S.W., Boden S.D. Neck pain: Medical diagnosis and comprehensive management. First edition, Philadelphia, WB Saunders Co. 1996.

Bridger R.S., Ossey S., Fourie G. Effect of lumbar traction on stature. Spine 1990;156:522-4.

Bulter D.S. Mobilisation of the Nervous System. First edition, Edinburgh, Churchill Livingstone 1991.

Cassidy J.D., Lopes A.A., Yong-Hing K. The immediate effect of manipulation versus mobilisation on pain and range of motion in cervical spine: A randomised controlled trial. J Manip Physiol Ther 1992;15:570-5.

Colachis S.C., Strohm B.R. A study of traction forces and angle of pull on vertebral interspaces in the cervical spine. Arch Phys Med Rehab 1965;46:820-30.

Cyriax J., Schitoz E.H. Manipulation past and present. London, William Heineman Ltd. 1975.

Deets D., Hands K.L., Hopp S.S. Cervical traction: a comparison of sitting and supine positions. Phys Ther 1977;57:255-61.

DeLarceda F.G. Effect of angle of traction pull on upper trapezius muscle activity. J Orthop Sports Phys Ther 1980;1:205-9.

Dwyer A., Aprill C., Bogduk N. Cervical zygapophyseal joint pain patterns I: A study in normal volunteers. Spine 1990;15:453-7.

Edwards B.C. Manual of Combined Movements. London, Churchill Livingstone 1992.

Gay R.E. The curve of the cervical spine: variations and significance. J Manip Physiol Ther 1993;16:591-4.

Goldie I., Landquist A. Evaluation of the effect of different forms of physiotherapy in cervical pain. Scand J Rehab Med 1970;2:117-21.

Gore D.R., Sepic S.B., Gardner G.M. Roentgenographic findings of the cervical spine in asymptomatic people. Spine 1986;11:521-4.

Grant R. Vertebral artery concerns: premanipulative testing of the cervical spine. Second edition, In: Grant R. ed, Physical therapy of the cervical and thoracic spine. New York, Churchill Livingstone Inc 1994.

Grieve G.P. Modern manual therapy of the vertebral column. Second edition, Edinburgh, Churchill Livingstone 1994.

Grimmer K. An investigation of poor cervical resting posture. Aust J Physiotherapy 1997;43:7-16.

Harris P.R. Cervical traction: review of literature and treatment guidelines. Phys Ther 1977;57:910-4.

Jette D.U., Falkel J.E., Trombly C. Effect of intermittent, supine cervical traction on the myoelectric activity of the upper trapezius muscle in subjects with neck pain. Phys Ther 1985;65:1173-6.

Jones H., Jones M., Maitland G.D. Examination and treatment by passive movement. Second edition, In: Grant R. ed, Physical therapy of the cervical and thoracic spine. New York, Churchill Livingstone Inc 1994.

Jones M. Clinical reasoning: The foundation of clinical practice. Part 1. Aust J Physiotherapy 1997;43:167-70.

Jones M.A. and Jones H.M. Principles of the physical examination. Second edition, In: Grieve G.P. ed, Modern manual therapy of the vertebral column. Edinburgh, Churchill Livingstone 1994.

Jones M.A. Clinical reasoning in manual therapy. Phys Ther 1992;72:875-84.

Jull G., Bodguk N., Marsland A. The accuracy of manual diagnosis for cervical zygapophyseal joint pain syndromes. Med J Aust 1988;148:233-6.

Jull G. Management of cervical headache. Manual Ther 1997;2:182-90.

Klaber-Moffett J.A., Hughes G.I., Griffiths P. An investigation of the effects of cervical traction. Part 1: clinical effectiveness. Clin Rehab 1990a;4:205-11.

Klaber-Moffett J.A., Hughes G.I., Griffiths P. An investigation of the effects of cervical traction. Part 2: the effects on the neck musculature. Clin Rehab 1990b;4:287-90.

Koes B.W., Assendelft W.J.J., van der Heijden G.J.M.G., Bouter L.M., Knipschild P.G. Spinal manipulation and mobilisation for back and neck pain. BMJ 1991;303:1298-303.

Koes B.W., Bouter L.M., van Mameren H., Essers A.H.M., Verstegen G.J.M.G., Hofhuizen D.M., Houben J.P., Knipschild P.G. Randomised clinical trial of manipulative therapy and physiotherapy for persistent back and neck complaints: Results of one year follow up. BMJ 1992;304:601-5.

Koes B.W., Bouter L.M., van Mameren H., Essers A.H.M., Verstegen G.J.M.G., Hofhuizen D.M., Houben J.P., Knipschild P.G. A randomised clinical trial of manual therapy and physiotherapy for persistent back and neck complaints: Subgroup analysis and relationship between outcome measures. J Manip Physiol Ther 1993;16:211-9.

Magarey M.E. Examination of the cervical and thoracic spine. Second edition, In: Grant R. ed, Physical therapy of the cervical and thoracic spine. New York, Churchill Livingstone Inc 1994.

Mahar C. Perception of stiffness in manipulative physiotherapy. Physiotherapy Theory and Practice 1995;11:35-44.

Mahar C., Adams R. Is the clinical concept of spinal stiffness multidimensional? Phys Ther 1995;75:854-64.

Maitland G.D. Vertebral Manipulation. Fifth edition, Boston, Butterworth 1986.

McCarthy M.R., O'Donoghue P.C., Yates C.K., Yates-McCarthy J.L. The clinical use of continuous passive motion in physical therapy. J Orthop Sports Phys Ther 1992;15:132-40.

McCarthy M.R., Yates C.K., Anderson M.A., Yates-McCarthy J.L. The effects of immediate continuous passive motion on pain during the inflammatory phase of soft tissue healing following anterior cruciate ligament reconstruction. J Orthop Sports Phys Ther 1993;17:96-101.

Murphy M.J. Effects of cervical traction on muscle activity. J Orthop Sports Phys Ther 1991:13:220-5.

O'Driscoll S.W., Kumar A., Salter R.B. The effect of continuous passive motion on the clearance of a haemarthrosis from a synovial joint. Clin Orthop 1983;176:305-11.

Ottenbacher K., Di Fabio R.P. Efficacy of spinal manipulation/mobilisation therapy: A meta-analysis. Spine 1985;10:833-7.

Peterson N.P., Vicenzino B., Wright A. The effects of a cervical mobilisation techniques on sympathetic outflow to the upper limb in normal subjects. Physiotherapy Theory and Practice 1993;9:149-56.

Saunders H.K. Use of spinal traction in the treatment of neck and back conditions. Clin Orthop 1983;179:31-8.

Slater H., Vicenzino B., Wright A. Sympathetic slump: the effects of novel manual therapy technique on peripheral sympathetic nervous system function. J Manual Manip Ther 1994;2:156-62.

Tan J.C., Nordin M. Role of physical therapy in the treatment of cervical disk disease. Orthop Clin North Am 1992;23:435-48.

Threlkeld A.J. The effects of manual therapy on connective tissue. Phys Ther 1992;72:893-902.

Trott P.H. Management of selected cervical syndromes. Second edition. In: Grant R. ed, Physical therapy of the cervical and thoracic spine. New York, Churchill Livingstone Inc 1994.

Van der Heijden G.J.M.G., Beurskens A.J.H.M., Koes B.W., Assendelft W.J.J., De Vet H.C.W., Bouter L.M. The efficacy of traction for back and neck pain: a systematic, blinded review of randomised clinical trial methods. Phys Ther 1995:75:93-104.

Vernon H.T., Aker P., Burns S., Viljakaanen S., Short L. Pressure pain threshold evaluation of the effect of spinal manipulation in the treatment of chronic neck pain: A pilot study. J Manip Physiol Ther 1990;13:13-6.

Vicenzino B., Collins D., Wright A. Sudomotor changes induced by neural mobilisation techniques in asymptomatic subjects. J Manual Manip Ther 1994;2:66-74.

Vicenzino B., Gutschalg F., Collins D., Wright A. An investigation of the effects of spinal manual therapy on forequarter pressure and thermal pain thresholds and sympathetic nervous system activity in asymptomatic subjects. In: Shacklock M. ed, Moving in on Pain. Melbourne, Butterworth Heinneman 1995:185-93.

Wright A. and Vicenzino B. Cervical mobilisation techniques, sympathetic nervous system effects and their relationship to analgesia. In: Shacklock M. ed, Moving in on Pain. Melbourne, Butterworth Heinneman 1995:164-73.

Wyke B.D. Articular neurology and manipulative therapy. In: Glasgow E.F. ed, Aspects of manipulative therapy. Edinburgh, Churchchill Livingstone 1985.

Zusman M., Edwards B., Donaghy A. Investigation of a proposed mechanism for the relief of spinal pain with passive joint movement. J Manual Med 1994;4:58-61.

Zylbergold R.S., Piper M.C. Cervical spine disorders: a comparison of three types of traction. Spine 1985;10:867-71.

Suggested reading list:

Borenstein D.G., Wiesel S.W., Boden S.D. Neck pain: Medical diagnosis and comprehensive management. First edition, Philadelphia, WB Saunders Co. 1996.

Grieve G.P. Modern manual therapy of the vertebral column. Second edition, Edinburgh, Churchill Livingstone 1994.

CHAPTER 16

VOCATIONAL REHABILITATION OF PATIENTS WITH CERVICAL SPINAL DISOREDERS

Cecilia W.P. Tsang-Li

WHAT IS VOCATIONAL REHABILITATION?

Vocational rehabilitation is a process of facilitation of optimal vocational development in individuals with disabilities through screening, evaluation, counselling, planning, training and placement, in order to help them to develop optimum vocational potential (Ellsworth *et al.*, 1980). The ultimate goals of vocational rehabilitation for people with disabilities are placement in competitive employment, personal satisfaction with the placement and satisfactory performance on the job through reduction or elimination of functional disabilities resulting from psychosocial, physical or developmental dysfunction (Robin & Roessler, 1995).

ROLES OF OCCUPATIONAL THERAPY IN VOCATIONAL REHABILITATION PROCESS

According to an official paper published in the American Journal of Occupational Therapy (Ellsworth *et al.*, 1980), the process of vocational rehabilitation can be subdivided into several stages.

Screening and evaluation

An initial interview is required to review the patient's occupational performance with regard to work, self-maintenance and leisure. This information is essential to identify the dysfunction of the patients. Further assessment of the patients' physical and functional performance may be required. Systematic evaluation should be planned according to the identified dysfunctions, in order to identify individual's capacity in different performance components, including assessment of strengths, motions, sensation, etc.

Treatment planning

Comprehensive treatment involves the use of selected activities, assistive devices and educational techniques to maximise the patients' independence in working, activities of daily living (ADL) and leisure. Such activities can also be used to improve work capacity, cognitive, social and emotional functions. Once the restorative phase of treatment is completed, the need for pre-vocational assessment will be considered.

Pre-vocational interest assessment and counselling

Therapists should identify their patients' vocational interests and goals, so that appropriate vocational interest tests can be given. Therapists and patients can then work together to explore the job opportunities that suit the patients' interests and capabilities. Patients with chronic pain often have fear returning to their previous job, as they may worry about the aggravation of pain from the job again. Careful consideration should be given to determine whether it is realistic to return to their previous jobs or to change to another jobs.

Pre-vocational evaluation

The goal of pre-vocational evaluation is to assess and predict the work behaviour and vocational potential of the patient through the application of practical, reality-based assessment techniques. Standardised work samples are commonly selected for pre-vocational evaluation.

Work adjustment services

Work adjustment involves a variety of tasks related to personal, social, daily living requirements, educational preparation and job readiness. This is often acquired through a well structured teaching learning programme. Therapists should monitor the psychological aspects of adjustment, particularly for those who cannot return to their previous jobs (Ellsworth *et al.*, 1980).

COMMON PROBLEMS FOR PATIETNS WITH NECK PAIN

Patients with cervical spinal injuries often complain of pain and stiffness (Ragnarsson, 1992). The pain is usually diffused throughout the neck, shoulder and suboccipital regions and can spread down to one or both arms. When symptoms are severe or do not stablise for weeks, further investigation, such as x-rays and other medical imaging, should be done. Chronic neck pain is often caused by high stress and demanding working environments. All symptoms and related information, such as onset, distribution, character, disease course and disturbance at work, should be carefully documented. Most patients with chronic pain will have complications, such as muscle atrophy and limited joint movements. Some patients may exhibit psychological problems and stress, especially when symptoms are related to work. Recurrence of symptoms is relatively common if the patient has insisted on continuing to work with the injury. It is well known that the longer the time period the patient is away from his job, the lower the chances are of him returning to work (Niemeyer *et al.*, 1993). It is therefore essential to start vocational rehabilitation for patients with cervical spinal disorders as early as possible.

VOCATIONAL REHABILITATION FOR PATIENTS WITH CERVICAL SPINAL DISORDERS

In work evaluation, occupational therapists will assist injured workers to develop work readiness and the necessary physical capacities (Holmes, 1985). Therapists will include work-oriented treatment in acute care setting, job analysis, work tolerance screening, work capacity evaluation, work hardening and job market re-entry management.

Work evaluation

Work evaluation is defined as a comprehensive process whereas real or simulated work will be used as a focal point for vocational assessment and exploration, which will be helpful for vocational development of individuals (Holmes, 1985). Medical, psychological, social, vocational, cultural and economic data can be incorporated to help injured workers to realise their highest level of functional independence.

Physical examination

The purposes of physical examination are to assess if patients are able to achieve the required physical functions, which will be essential for the participation in work evaluation. It is also essential to identify the presence of abnormal behaviour and to provide baseline information about the neuromuscular system (Matheson, 1997). Prior to the physical assessment, data on the patients' medical history and present medical conditions should be assessed. Specific complaints should be documented and the results of relevant medical investigations should be recorded. This information will provide a thorough understanding of the patient's medical status. Assessment should also include the patient's job history, job demands and the nature of the injuries that affect the physical functions. Therapists should not forget to assess patient's own perception of his disabilities and his views towards a future vocational plan. Objective evaluation should include assessment of posture, anthropometry, vertigo, shoulder protraction and retraction in sitting. Using an inclinometer and goniometers, assessment of the range of motion of the joins at cervical region, the shoulder and the elbow are essential. The muscle strength of the neck, shoulder, elbow, wrist, thumb and finger should also be tested (Figure 1). A comprehensive sensory test of various dermatomes is important because neurological signs related to nerve compression should be assessed.

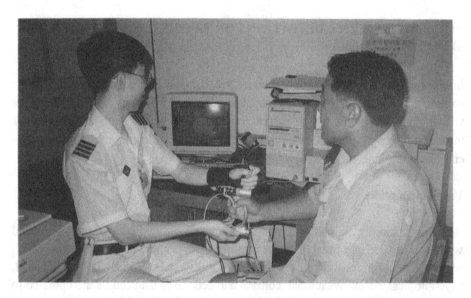

Figure 1. Dexter hand evaluation system to measure grip strength and endurance.

Work capacity evaluation

Neck injuries are frequently associated with jobs involving repetitive motion in the shoulders and neck, particularly when prolonged static sitting or standing working posture is required. Therefore, therapists should be prepared to understand various types of work samples that simulates or resemble either sedentary or manual work (Figure 2). Common work samples used for patients with cervical spinal disorders are listed in Table 1.

Table 1. Common work samples for evaluation of patients with cervical disorders.

Valpar 4:	Upper extremity range of motion
Valpar 5:	Clerical comprehension and aptitude
Valpar 9:	Whole body range of motion
Valpar 19:	Dynamic physical capacity

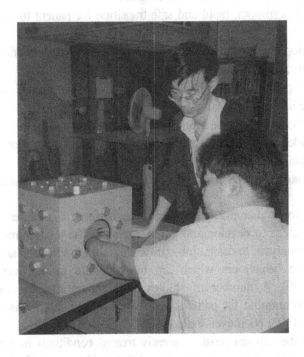

Figure 2. Valpar work samples are common work evaluation tools to evaluate work capacity. This Valpar work sample 4 can be used to assess upper extremity range of motion.

The BTE Primus and the LIDO work simulator are common equipment which can simulate various work situations so as to assess work capacity. The work cube, WEST system and Key work hardening system are often used in the assessment of work capacity and for work hardening. When administering different work samples, therapists should refer to appropriate operational manuals so that assessment procedures can be standardised. Comparison of results between patients and normative data is then possible. The reliability and validity of the prediction power of these evaluations can then be maintained.

Work hardening

Work hardening is a structured, productivity oriented programme, using real or simulated activities, which can serve as a treatment with the ultimate goal of assisting clients to achieve a level of productivity that is acceptable in the labour market (AOTA, 1989; King, 1993). It has been also defined by the Commission on Accreditation of Rehabilitation Facilities (CARF, 1991) as graded conditioned tasks which can progressively improve the biomechanical, neuromuscular, cardiovascular or metabolic and psychosocial functions of the patient. Work hardening can help to bridge the gap between acute care and returning to work (Key, 1991). The goals of work hardening are:

a. to ensure a smooth, rapid and safe transition for patient to return to the work force,
b. to develop the physical condition of patients towards work, including their flexibility, strength and stamina,
c. to develop safe working habits, such as correct sitting and standing postures and safe lifting practices,
d. to develop and reinforce appropriate worker behaviours,
e. to provide an objective measurement of the worker's physical tolerance, which is essential to prepare for their vocational planning and
f. to evaluate the effectiveness of new tools or job site modifications.

Occupational therapists are trained to perform a number of work-related activities, such as to develop and guide a job-specific programme for workers, to perform job analysis, to design job station and tool modification and to identify and remedy those behaviours which are inappropriate in the work environment. (AOTA, 1989). A number of studies have shown that the value of a work hardening programme for patients with work-related injuries is great (Callahan, 1992; King, 1993; Niemeyer *et al.*, 1993).

Among the top ten most frequently treated conditions in a work hardening programme, 14% of the patients suffered from either cervical, shoulder or rotator cuff injuries (King, 1993). Nearly 50% of the patients returned to their previous job and 30.5% had changed or modified their jobs and 13.6% were referred to vocational counselling services (Niemeyer *et al.*, 1993).

It was also found that as the duration of disability increased, the chances of returning to work decreased significantly. In Hong Kong, simulated work environments are usually set up in occupational therapy unit to provide the work hardening programme (Figure 3). New equipment, like the BTE Primus, Lido work simulator and Valpar work components, are commonly used for work hardening.

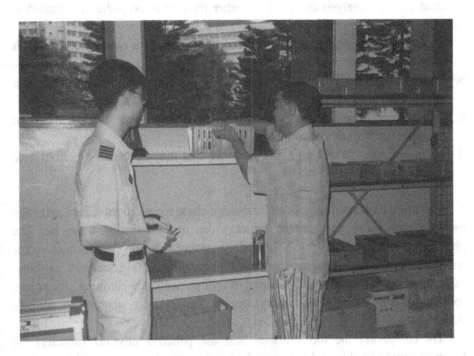

Figure 3. A work hardening programme for a patient with chronic neck pain and the treatment aim is to simulate frequent lifting of heavy objects at various heights.

Patients who suffer from cervical pain may be either a sedentary worker requiring prolonged static posture, e.g. a keyboard operator, or a manual labourer who has a lot of upper body motion in the course of his work, e.g. construction site worker, cook. Due to the diversity of patients' backgrounds, a comprehensive work hardening programme should be planned to accommodate the demands of different types of work. Detailed job analysis, including a visit to the job site, is a prerequisite of an effective work hardening programme.

Job analysis and job matching

It is important to ensure that job demands and the worker's functional capacities are matched. By careful job analysis, therapists can assess the physical demands of work tasks required and the functional capacities of the injured worker. Vocational goals can then be planned to decide whether workers can return to their previous jobs independently or if modifications of the job tasks are necessary to keep the worker in the same job. In most of the cases, therapists may need to modify the workers' working habits or physical capacity. For example, patients may need to change their work habits, work posture, work tools ...etc. in order to return to work successfully. Job analysis can be done either through a comprehensive interview with the injured worker or a job site visit. The purposes are:

a. to assess the nature of a job for the development of a comprehensive work hardening programme,

b. to investigate the difference between an injured worker's functional abilities and his job tasks demands,

c. to recommend any necessary modifications in equipment or work habits to enhance the worker's performance,

d. to assess other factors, e.g. specific tools, that may affect work performance (Matheson, 1997).

Common tools used for job site analysis include force gauges (Chatillon), tape measure, stop watch, lap counter, camera/video recorder, inclinometer, etc. The physical demands of the job, including sitting, standing, reaching, motor coordination, medium dexterity, resistive tool handling, lifting, carrying, pushing, pulling, stooping, kneeling, crouching, crawling, walking, climbing, balancing, foot or hand controls, visual acuity, talking, hearing and vibration, should be documented.

By comparing the job demands and the patient's physical capacity, the therapist should be able to determine whether the patient can return to his previous job or whether modifications of the working equipment are required. Treatment can be then directed towards improving the worker's physical capacity by adopting correct postures or body mechanics. Sometimes, the affected area can be immobilised, with an appropriate appliance or supportive device to reduce pain during certain work motions.

If all these methods are unsuccessful, therapists may then need to consider job matching and job placement with the assistance of other disciplines, such as social workers, psychologists or rehabilitation counsellors.

CASE STUDY

Mr. Wong was a 56-year-old cook who was working for people with sever physical handicaps at a workshop. He had suffered from work-related right clavicle and neck pain. Radiographs did not show any abnormalities on his cervical spine, except some degenerative signs at the C7 level. After his initial medical consultation, he was given some analgesics and seven days sick leave. Since then, his pain gradually subsided and Mr Wong then resumed his work. A few days later, his pain, however, became severe again, especially after work. He then consulted an orthopaedic surgeon and was referred to occupational therapy for vocational evaluation and rehabilitation. Initial assessment was then done.

It was found that Mr. Wong had limited neck rotation and lateral flexion. The restriction of movement was more series on the left side than on the right side. He complained of severe pain on the left-hand side of his neck near the scapula with a visual analogue scale (VAS) score of 6.5. From the initial interview, Mr. Wong lived with his wife and three children in a resettlement estate, near his work place. His eldest son had just enrolled in a local university and the other two children were currently studying in secondary schools. As he was the only breadwinner in the family, he continued to work despite knowing that his job was very physically demanding. Physical capacity evaluation was done using the LIDO work simulator, the Dexter hand evaluation system and the Valpar component 19. It was found that Mr. Wong's grip deteriorated in his left hand and left upper limb, which was probably due to pain. The strength of the grip his right hand was normal as compared with other people of his age. He was able to lift 10lbs. weight. Mr. Wong reported that he had to purchase a lot of food every morning and then cook two meals for the mentally handicapped residents in the workshop. He brings a trolley and uses it to carry the food from market. But as soon as he completed cooking the meal, he felt general fatigue and pain on the left shoulder. Then, a long break was needed before he was able to cook dinner. On examination of his work history, Mr. Wong used to work in large restaurants and had to work shift duties. He found that his health was deteriorating as he gained weight. He therefore changed his job and worked at his current position, as he thought the work might be less demanding. He worked in this capacity for one year. A few months before the interview, one of his colleagues resigned and he therefore had to take up his partner's job. Due to budget constraints, his partner's position was not filled. His neck pain seemed to be associated with the increase in workload. A visit was made to his workplace, with the aims of investigating Mr Wong's work demands and his working habits. During this visit, therapists measured the force required for pushing and pulling the trolley using a Chaterllon Force Measurement Gauge (Figure 4). The significant findings of the visit are listed as follows:

1. The height of his working tables and stoves were too high and Mr. Wong had to elevate his arms to prepare the food.
2. The general work demands in the kitchen were high. On average, Mr. Wong needed to lift about 30lbs. food and to pull or push about 80 lbs. of food on trolley.
3. The ergonomic design of the kitchen was not good. Most of the materials had been put on a workbench, which was at a distance away from the stove. Mr. Wong had to twist his body and stretch his left hand to get the desired materials while his right hand was required to hold a heavy frying pan. These work demands were found to cause strain to the neck extensor, the shoulder and the elbow of the left upper limb.

4. When Mr. Wong was cooking or preparing food, there was a tendency to laterally flex of his neck towards the left side. This was probably because he had to lift the heavy frying pan using his right hand. It could be due to the deterioration of muscle strength on his right hand that he then tried to compensate through lateral flexion of the neck and trunk.

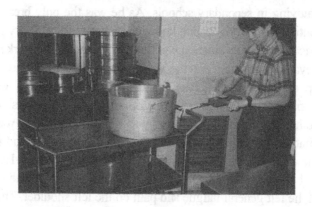

Figure 4. Measurment of the force required for pushing and pulling the trolley using a Chaterllon Force Measurement Gauage.

After the assessment of work demands and work capacity evaluation, a comprehensive vocational rehabilitation programme was planned. A work hardening programme was designed to assist Mr. Wong to return to his job. The programme included:
a. Valpar 19 to simulate food lifting in the kitchen,
b. LIDO work simulator with an adapted handle to simulate frying activities (Figure 5),
c. BTE primus to simulate push/pull of heavy goods.

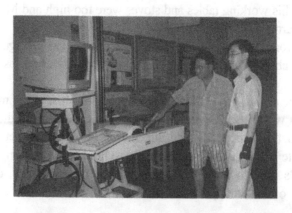

Figure 5. Work hardening programme using LIDO work to simulate frying activities.

Education of correct working postures

In the work hardening programme, Mr. Wong was educated on how to correctly lift and transfer on heavy objects, and the proper standing posture for cooking (Figure 6). Mr. Wong's work posture was further assessed using a video recorder. The results were discussed with him to provide visual feedback of his performance. Mr. Wong soon realised that his neck pain was mainly due to improper lateral flexion of his neck. He was also taught various energy conservation techniques that could be used during work. The importance of regular rest between work activities was stressed.

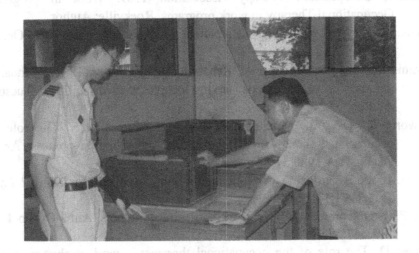

Figure 6. Simulated work training programme in an occupational therapy unit to teach correct posture at work (pulling the trolley of food around the kitchen).

Improvement in physical capacity

Training of grip strength and general upper limb strength were emphasised. The BTE primus was employed to strengthen his grip, the general muscle power of both upper limbs and to build up his endurance for standing by adopting the correct posture.

Ergonomic of the work site

As the working bench was found too far away from the stove, it was recommended that it should be moved closer so that Mr. Wong could reach the food easily. It was also recommended that the height of the working bench and the stove be lowered. Unnecessary shoulder elevation at work can thus be avoided. Unfortunately, these recommendations were rejected by the management of the workshop, due to financial constraints. Mr. Wong had resumed his job after joining this comprehensive treatment programme. His pain level decreased below 2 for the VAS, although occasional tightness and fatigue of the neck muscles were reported. In a follow up visit, Mr. Wong found mild tenderness and stiffness on the left side of his neck and clavicle. However, he managed to cope with his work without aggravating his neck pain. Eventually he successfully re-adjusted to his work place.

References:

American Occupational Therapy Association 1989. Work in progress: Occupational Therapy in work programs. Rockville: Author.

Callahan D.K. Work Hardening for a patient with low back pain. Am J Occup Ther 1992;47:645-9.

Commission on Accreditation of Rehabilitation Facilities 1991. Standards manual for organizations serving people with disabilities. Tucson: Author.

Ellsworth P., Davy J., Mitcham M., Parkin J., Presseller S. The role of occupational therapy in the vocational rehabilitation process. Am J Occup Ther 1980;31:881-3.

Key G.L. Work hardening or work conditioning: semantic or reality? Phys Ther 1991;14:12-6.

King P.M. Outcome analysis of work-hardening programs. Am J Occup Ther 1993;47:595-603.

Holmes D. The role of the occupational therapist – work evaluator. Am J Occup Ther 1985;39:308-13.

Matheson R. The 1997 Industrial Rehabilitation Professional Residency. Keele, NH 1997.

Niemeyer L.O., Jacobs K., Reynolds-Lynch K., Bettencourt C., Lang S. Work hardening: past, present, and future – The work programs special interest section national work hardening outcome study. Am J Occup Ther 1993;48:327-39.

Ragnarsson K.T. Rehabilitation of patients with cervical spine disorders. In: Camins M.B. and O'Leary P.F. eds, Disorders of the Cervical Spine. Baltimore, Williams & Wilkins 1992:337-51.

Robin S.E., Roessler R.T. Foundations of the Vocational Rehabilitation Process. Fourth edition, Texas, Pro-ed 1995.

CHAPTER 17

COMMUNITY EDUCATION ON NECK CARE

Hon Sun Lai

INTRODUCTION

The cost of healthcare is one of the major expenditures in most countries
(OECD, 1994). Moreover, it has been growing rapidly in recent years and
governments of different countries have tried to search for the best ways to
provide efficient and effective health services (Abel-Smith, 1994; Redmand,
1993). It has been recognised that health education is an integral part of safe
and cost-effective means of patient management. Heinrick *et al.* (1985) suggest
that it is possible to prevent, promote, maintain, or modify a number of health
related behaviours by educating patients on their illnesses. Musculoskeletal
problems, such as cervical disorders, whiplash injuries, stress-related diseases
and work-related injuries, are common orthopaedic conditions requiring
medical treatment and take up a large portion of the health budget (Reid,
1996). Most recurrent injuries can be prevented if patients have a better
understanding of the disorders and body awareness (Hayne, 1988).
Physiotherapists are concerned with both treatment and prevention of neck
conditions. They are also in a unique position to provide patients with
information which may help to prevent the recurrence of neck disorders and
thus reduce healthcare costs (Sluijs, 1991).

NECK CARE EDUCATION

Neck care education is a communication process between physiotherapists and
patients. Physiotherapists may use a combination of methods, such as
teaching, counselling and behaviour modification techniques, to promote a
patient's knowledge and understanding of health (Hamilton-Duckett and Kidd,
1985; Bartlett, 1985). Research shows that behaviour therapy programmes for
chronic pain can effectively lengthen the period of symptom relief (Cinciripin

and Floreen 1982; Roberts and Reinhart, 1980). Although a number of studies have reported the efficacy of conservative treatment for neck pain (Gross *et al.*, 1996; Friedrich *et al.*, 1996), cervical spinal disorders treated by physiotherapists often show a high recurrence rate. However, this can be controlled or even avoided by educating patients with appropriate preventive measures (Saunders and Maxwell, 1988; Leathley, 1988). Fisk *et al.* (1983) believe that if people are equipped with the right information, they can build up their self-confidence and effectively adjust and manage their neck conditions.

DEVELOPING NECK CARE EDUCATION PROGRAMMES

With neck care education, physiotherapists should encourage patients to take up their advice and follow instructions in order to prevent recurrence of injuries (Sluijs, 1991). The education programme can be non-specific and provide some general information about neck care for the public. Conversely, it can be designed for a specific target group such as computer operators, office workers, manual workers or school children. In order to develop an effective programme, physiotherapists should explore the characteristics of the target group and then design an education programme which can meet the target group's needs (Hayne, 1988). Physiotherapists should follow a four-step process, including assessment, planning, implementation and evaluation, in developing a neck care education programme (Figure 1).

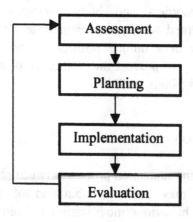

Figure 1. The process of the development of a health education programme.

ASSESSMENT

Assessment is the first step in developing a patient education programme (Lorig, 1977). It is a systematic data collection process to identify the needs and problems of patients (Schultz *et al.*, 1988; Rankin and Stallings, 1990). Physiotherapists can then use this information to plan, implement and evaluate an effective education programme. This assessment procedure will be useful to avoid providing patients with unnecessary or repeated information. It will also be useful to remind therapists to present their information at a patients' level of understanding (Smith, 1987). For example, patients with chronic neck pain will demand for more information about self-management of pain and about adaptation of lifestyle to cope with pain. Office workers may demand for information related to ergonomics so that they can help themselves to avoid occupational neck problems. Patient compliance is one of the major factors determining the success of a health education programme. Compliance in medicine has been defined as the degree to which a patient adheres to a prescribed regimen (Ice, 1985). When the information provided to patients cannot satisfy their needs, it may cause non-compliance. During assessment, physiotherapists should determine the characteristics of the target group. Three common aspects should be assessed, including the patients' patho-physiological, socio-demographic and psychological backgrounds (Magora, 1973; Nagi *et al.*, 1973; Mayo, 1978).

Pathophysiological factors

Through assessment, therapists should determine what kind of neck disorders the patients are suffering from. Therapists should also have a good understanding of the disease involved (e.g. acute or chronic), the prognosis and aggravating factors. It is important to check what patients already know so that the content of the programme can build upon their knowledge level. Unnecessary duplication of information can be avoided (Hough, 1987; May, 1983). Simth (1987) pointed out that the physical effects of a particular condition, such as pain or discomfort, can diminish the ability of a person to concentrate on the information he or she is receiving. Therefore, one should bear this in mind in planning the venue, time and duration of the education session.

Socio-demographic factors

The socio-demographic variables are individual characteristics such as age, sex, education, occupation, income, marital status and religion, which can affect the understanding and compliance of neck care instructions and exercise regimes (Rankin and Stallings, 1990). If the patients are either very young or very old, they may have a higher non-compliance rate and difficulties in understanding the presentation content (Bergman and Werner, 1963, Schwartz, *et al.*, 1962). Extreme socio-economic or occupational status was found to affect compliance negatively (Mayo, 1978).

Psychological factors

Psychological factors may determine patients' general behaviour and can thus affect whether they comply to instructions. The most common psychological factors influencing patients' behaviour are their perceptions, motives, attitudes and personalities (Becker and Mailman, 1975). If patients find that the information provided is not helpful, they will not be motivated to perform neck exercises or follow any instructions. In addition, Becker and Mailman (1975) further pointed out that the attitude towards illness, treatment and pain can affect patients' compliance. Sometimes, modifications of the programme are required to fit "individual traits".

PLANNING

In planning a neck care education programme, specific objectives must be established (Smith, 1987). Due to limited resources, physiotherapists should make learning objectives specific, measurable and attainable (Hayne, 1988). In general, the objectives of teaching are to promote knowledge, improve attitudes, develop skills and enhance perceptual abilities. Education programme planning should also make use of learning psychology principles, such as knowledge, attitude and psychomotor (Redmand, 1993; Smith, 1987).

Knowledge

Objectives referring to knowledge are often regarded as cognitive. In cognitive theory, learning is the development of insights or understanding that provide a potential guide for behaviour (Redman, 1993). Based on this theory, therapists should organise the content of a neck care programme so that it can be easily assimilated by patients. If the objectives are too ambitious, patients may be overloaded with information which may lead to misunderstanding or loss of interest by the patients in carrying out the given instructions (May, 1983). In neck care education programmes, therapists usually cover many topics, including the anatomy of the cervical spine, the patho-physiology of selected neck conditions specific to the target group, posture re-education instructions and neck exercises. Other specific information, such as ergonomic skills and home environment settings are provided to office workers and housewives respectively. Altogether there are many types of information which may be of interest to patients. Thus, presenting a large amount of information in a logical and succinct manner is not easy, especially when presentation time is limited and patients often have short attention spans.

Attitude

An attitude is a learned, emotionally tuned pre-disposition to react in a particular way towards an object or an idea (Klausmeirer, 1985). Patients' attitudes towards their conditions may determine how well they will receive the information in the education programme and comply with the given instructions. It was found that education programmes are of limited value if patients do not change their attitude and motivation (Korhonen *et al.*, 1983). Thus, therapists should develop programme objectives to pinpoint patients' attitudes towards their neck problems and how they can make changes in their lifestyles or daily activities.

Psychomotor

Objectives outlining skills may be regarded as psychomotor. To perform a particular skill, a person must possess both a healthy neuromotor system and the ability to form a mental image of the act (Redmand, 1993). In teaching correct postures and exercises, it is important to use visual illustrations and demonstrations to help the patients to develop mental images of the acts. It is recommended that demonstration and self practice will help patients to retain the mental images of new exercises or posture more effectively (Simth, 1987). However, practice periods should be short and regular, but not too frequent to cause fatigue (Klausmeirer, 1985).

IMPLEMENTATION

Having developed the learning objectives, the therapist will then implement the education plan for the target group. The instructions and teaching methods will be based on the information gathered in the assessment and planning. Factors such as patients' needs, level of anxiety and amount of time available for the learning should also be considered (Dickson and Maxwell, 1985; Redmand, 1993). Therapists should encourage patients to use the information provided to manage their own health situation. For success of the behavioural education, emphasis should be placed on self-care behaviour such as performing regular neck exercises, postural re-education, and/or adjustment of working environment or posture. Most therapists have a tendency to over-estimate the compliance of their audience (Wagstaff, 1982) and provide too much information in each presentation. If the audience misunderstand the information provided, they may carry out the instructions wrongly or not carry them out at all (Ley, 1977). Therefore, the information provided should be precise and specific. Information should be given in a simple and direct way so that the audience can follow the instructions. If necessary, important messages should be emphasised repeatedly (Kindelan and Kent, 1986). Neck care education can be carried out in different ways, such as advice after treatment sessions, neck care brochures, posters, videos and neck care seminars. Therapists should consider the patients' characteristics (patho-physiological, socioeconomic and psychological), the availability of resources, such as time constraints or funding available, as well as the specific needs of particular patient groups. Computer technology can also be used to present information through computer programmes or the Internet (Redmand, 1993). The following are some examples of different forms of neck care education.

(1) Advice

Advice is usually given by therapists on a one-to-one basis after a treatment session (Schultz *et al.*, 1988). Therapists can also demonstrate correct neck exercises or posture to patients directly. It may be the most effective way educating the patients. Such advice will be given according to individual conditions or problems. However, the information given will be limited and this method may not be efficient when therapist have to educate a number of patients.

(2) Posters and pamphlets

Both posters and pamphlets are good teaching materials in neck care education (Rankin and Stalling, 1990). The poster can be displayed on notice boards or in public access areas. However, the information that can be put on each poster will be limited. Therefore, the message included should be simple and direct, highlighting the most important points. As compared with posters, pamphlets can contain more information. Patients can pick up a pamphlet and read it at home. With pamphlets, patients can read them at their own leisure and this will promote their understanding of the given information. However, the information included is limited and the production cost of pamphlets may be relatively expensive. Therefore, posters and pamphlets are mainly used to provide general information for the public or the local communities.

(3) Group seminars

Seminars can be designed to accommodate the needs of a particular group of people. This encourages active interaction between the presenter and the audience. The number of participants should be limited so that the interaction is under control. In preparing for neck care education seminars, a few points should be noted because they can help to make the seminar interesting. Instead of using a classic lecture style, the presenter can use other teaching methods, such as small group discussion, problem-solving of case presentations to encourage active participation by the audience. These activities will encourage the audience to be active participants rather than passive listeners. Patients may find these experiences more personal and interesting. Long term learning effects are thus made possible. When the anatomy and pathology of neck conditions are presented, various forms of audio-visual aids including anatomical models, videotapes, posters, computer-aided presentations, can be used to provide visual illustrations. A good combination of different presentation aids and group activities will help to hold participants' interest and attention. It is also very important to explain the purpose and outline of the presentation content at the beginning of each session so that the audience is prepared for it. At the end of the session, it is useful to have a summary of the content covered and to allow some time for questions and answers.

(4) Video recording

Video recording is an effective form of presentation. It can present vivid, illustrative materials which are difficult to be described by other means (Redmand, 1993). Video recording can also be employed to present experiences, places and situations that can simulate real life situations and help patients to change their attitude and develop an understanding. It assists the audience to develop mental images of appropriate ways of doing exercises and will be particularly effective for patients with limited reading abilities. However, video recording does not interact with the audience. Production costs can also be very expensive.

(5) Computer aided programmes or Internet Webpages

With modern technology, people have greater access to information through computer aided programmes or Internet Webpages. There are many resources available for patients to learn about neck disorders and how to correctly perform neck exercises and to correct their posture. There are six types of computer assisted instructions: drill and practice, tutorials, problem solving, simulation, gaming and testing (Rankin and Stallings, 1990). These programmed instructions take advantage of learning principles that cannot be facilitated in other teaching techniques, particularly for large groups of learners. In this method, patients are required to be active learners. The computer can provide immediate feedback, correct wrong answers and reinforce correct answers. Relevant and most updated information can also be circulated through Internet Webpages. Patients can then browse through relevant information in their leisure time.

FEEDBACK

Evaluation is a vital part of the patient education process, whether in the teaching process of an individual patient or in the development of an effective patient education programme (Smith, 1987). Through evaluation exercises, therapists can assess the effectiveness of their programmes (Smith, 1987). The results of the evaluation can also assist therapists to optimise the outcome under the constraints of limited resources. Unfortunately, evaluation is often neglected by therapists.

As evaluation will be performed based on the programme objectives, if the objectives have been clearly defined, evaluation will be a straightforward exercise. Evaluation can be performed to assess either the individual's progress or the neck care education programme as a whole. Individual evaluation is commonly performed to determine the progress of individual patients in achieving the established objectives (Redmand, 1993). This type of evaluation is done by checking if the patient can perform his neck exercises correctly or if there is improvement in his posture. Programme evaluation is commonly performed to assess if a neck care education programme functions effectively or if the participants are able to achieve the objectives. Once the objectives of evaluation have been decided, careful planning is necessary to identify what is meaningful in the assessment, what essential data must be collected and what resources are required. Evaluation planning involves two important elements, which are known as focusing and designing. Focusing is a procedure to define the audience, purpose and scope of evaluation, to delineate specific questions and to assess any available resources. Designing involves the construction of instruments to collect data. There are many different types of evaluation methods and readers are encouraged to refer to the literature (Rankin and Stallings, 1990; Redmand, 1993).

Direct observation

Therapists can observe patients doing specific neck exercises or postures that have been taught. This kind of evaluation can provide accurate and descriptive data (Rankin and Stallings, 1990). Patients should receive immediate feedback and guidance to reinforce their learning.

Questionnaires

Questionnaires with either open or closed response formats can be used to collect patients' feedback. Open-ended questions will encourage respondents to express themselves as much as they want. However, data are difficult to tabulate and analyse (Rankin and Stalling, 1990). Close-ended questions involve scaled, ranked, yes/no, multiple choice, fill-in blank or checklist responses. Questionnaires must be carefully designed and validated before formal implementation. Ambiguous questions, unclear instructions and errors must be corrected.

Interviews

Interviews are also effective for collecting patients' feedback. The response rate is normally high. It can either be in an unstructured or structured questionnaire format. The disadvantages of conducting interviews are that the process can be time consuming and patients' responses can be biased by inexperienced interviewers.

SUMMARY

Neck disorders and diseases treated by therapists often show a high rate of recurrence. Neck care education is an integral part of physiotherapy in the management of neck disorders. The development of a neck care programme can be done by following a four-step process, including assessment, planning, implementation and evaluation. Neck care education programmes should be structured to meet the specific needs of patients or the community. The aim of the programme is to promote the knowledge of the patient, prevent recurrence of injuries and reduce healthcare expenditure.

References:

Abel-Smith B. In Chapter 11: Public health expenditure and the economic crisis, in an introduction to health: Policy, planning, and financing. New York, Longman Publishing 1994:149-63.

Bartlett E.E. At last, a definition. Patient education and counselling 1985; 7:323-324.

Becker M., Mailman L. Socio-behavioral determinants of compliance and medical care recommendation. Med Care 1975; 13:10-24.

Bergman A.B., Werner R.J. Failure of Children to receive penicillin by mouth. N Engl J Med 1963;268:1334-8.

Dickson D.A. and Maxwell M. The interpersonal dimension of physiotherapy: implications for training. Physiotherapy 1985;71:306-10.

Cinciripini P., Floreen A. An evaluation of a behavioral programme for chronic pain. J Behavioral Med 1982;5:376-89.

Fisk D., Dimonte A., Courington G. Implementation of educational programs for patients. Nurs Admin Quart 1983;8:61-5.

Friedrich M., Cermak T., Maderbacher P. The effect of brochure use versus therapist teaching on patients performing therapeutic exercises and on changes in impairment status. Phys Ther 1996;76:1082-8.

Gross A.R., Aker P.D., Goldsmith C.H., Peloso P. Conservative management of mechanical neck disorders. A systemic overview and meta-analysis. Online Journal of Current Clinical Trials 1996;30:200-1.

Hamilton-Duckett P., Kidd L. Counselling skill and the physiotherapist. Physiotherapy. 1985;71:179-80.

Hayne C.R. The preventive role of physiotherapy in the national health service and industry. Physiotherapy 1988;74:2-3.

Heinrick R., Cohen M., Naiboff B., Collins G., Bonebakker A. Comparing physical and behaviour therapy for chronic low back pain on physical abilities, psychological distress and patient's perceptions. J Behavioral Med 1985,8:61-78.

Hough A. Communication in healthcare. Physiotherapy. 1987;73:56-59.

Ice R. Long term compliance. Phys Ther 1985;65:1832-9.

Kindelan K., Kent G. Patients' preferences for information. J Royal College General Prac 1986; 36:461-3.

Klausmeier H.J. Education psychology. Fifth edition, New York, Harper and Row 1985.

Korhonen A., Guccione A, DeMonte F. Interpersonal skills education in entry level physical therapy program. Phys Ther 1983;63:388-93.

Leathley M. Physiotherapy and health education: report of a survey. Physiotherapy 1988; 74:218-20.

Ley P. Communicating with the patient, in introductory psychology: a textbook for health students. London, Routledge and Kegan 1977.

Lorig K. An overview of needs assessments tools for continuing education. Nurse Educator 1977;3:12-6.

Magora A. Investigation of the relation between low back pain and occupation. Scand J Rehabil Med 1973;7:146.

May B.J. Teaching: a skill in clinical practice. Phys Ther 1983; 63:1627-33.

Mayo N.E. Patient compliance-practical implication for physical therapist: a review of literature. Phys Ther 1978;58:1083-90.

Nagi A.D., Riely K.A., Newby P. The health believe moedl and behviour related to chronic illness. Health Edu Quart 1973;6:1-47.

Norton S. Support for physiotherapist in health education. Physiotherapy 1986;82:5-7.

OECD (Organisation for Economic Cooperation and Development). In Chapter 1: The reform of healthcare system: A review of seventeen OECD countries. Paris, OECD 1994:11-14.

Rankin S.H., Stalling K.D. Patient education: issues, principle and practices. Philadelphia, JB Lippincott Company 1990.

Redmand B.K. The process of patient education. Seventh edition, St Louis, Mosby Year Book 1993.

Reid A. Amount of patient education in physical therapy practice and perceived effects. Phys Ther 1996;76:1089-96.

Roberts A., Reinhart L. The behavioral management of chronic pain: long term follow-up with comparison groups. Pain 1980;8:151-62.

Saunders C., Maxwell M. The case for counselling in physiotherapy. Physiotherapy 1988;74:592-5.

Schultz C.L., Wellard R., Swerissen H. Communication and interpersonal helping skills: an essential component in physiotherapy education? Aust Physiotherapy Assoc 1988;34:75-80.

Schwartz D., Wang M., Zeitz L. Medication errors made by elderly, chronically ill patient. Am J Pub Health 1962;52:2018-29.

Smith C.E. Patient education: nurses in partnership with other health professions. Philadephia, WB Saunders Company 1987.

Sluijis M.E. A checklist to assess patient ediuation in physical therapy practice: Development and reliability. Phys Ther 1991;71:561-8.

Wagstaff G.F. A small dose of commonsense-communication, persuasion and physiotherapy. Physiotherapy 1982;68: 327-9.

Suggested reading list:

Aronson E. The social animal, in Social psychology. San Franscio, Freeman 1977.

Bradshaw P.W., Kinsey J.A., Ley P., Bradshaw J. Recall of medical advice, comprehensibility an specificity. Br J Soc Clin Psy 1975;14:5-62.

Ellencweig A.U. In Chapter 2: Health systems-a critical analysis of existing and suggested model. In analysing health system. A modular approach. New York, Oxford University Press 1992:16-42.

Hayne C.R. Back schools and total back care programmes-a review. Physiotherapy 1984;70:14.

Liston C.B. Back Schools and Ergonomics. In physical therapy of the low back pain. New York, Churchill Livingstone 1987.

Lyne P.A. The professions allied to Medicine. Physiotherapy 1986;72:8-10.

Versloot J.M., Rozeman A., Van Son A.M., Van Akkerveeken .PF. The cost effectiveness of back school programme in industry, a longitudinal controlled field study. Spine 1992;12: 22-7.

PART V

Advanced Studies in
Cervical Spinal Disorders

CHAPTER 18

CURRENT RESEARCH IN NECK PAIN AND ITS REHABILITATION

Sai Wing Lee

INTRODUCTION

Despite the fact that cervical spinal disorders are relatively common in the general population, our understanding of these conditions remain limited. Further investigation in this field is therefore necessary. These investigations will be helpful in improving our confidence in making diagnosis for patients. Treatment effectiveness can then be improved. Recurrence of cervical spinal disorders can also be minimised.

Current research on cervical spinal disorders can generally be divided into different areas, including bone and joints of the cervical spine, physiological functions of neck muscles, neurology of the cervical spine, cervical intervertebral disc, traumatology of the neck, diagnostic imaging techniques, surgical and non-surgical treatment for cervical disorders, epidemiology and work-related cervical spinal disorders. Some recent development in these areas will be introduced in the following subsections.

BONE AND JOINTS OF THE CERVICAL SPINE

As some age-old problems in cervical spinal disorders remain unresolved while new clinical problems emerge, it is necessary to revisit some of the basic sciences of the cervical spine. Investigation of the bones and joints of the cervical spine provides valuable information for the assessment and treatment of patients with cervical spinal disorders. For example, Panjabi *et al.* (1993) have investigated the three-dimensional anatomy of the facet joints in the spine, using 12 fresh autopsy specimens. The orientation of the facet joints have been assessed and quantified. Anatomical differences in the facet joints of the cervical, thoracic and lumbar regions have been compared. Further studies in the biomechanics of the cervical spine are then possible. With the advancement of computer technologies, Yoganandan *et al.* (1996) have developed a model of the human cervical spine using finite element technology. This type of computer modelling is not only useful to understand the kinematics of the cervical spine, but is also useful to investigate the mechanical effects of trauma and new surgical interventions, particularly as these interventions cannot be performed in *in vivo*.

NECK MUSCLES

Muscles are the active driving forces for producing head and neck motion and for protecting the cervical spine. As compared with those of the thoracic and lumbar spine, the sizes of cervical muscles are relatively small and their alignment is complicated. These anatomical arrangements suggest that fine control of the head and neck motion is required. However, the interactions of cervical spinal muscles, or even the basic anatomical functions of some deep neck muscles, remain unclear. Further investigation of cervical spinal muscles is therefore required.

Mayoux-Benhamou *et al.* (1994) have investigated the morphometry of longus colli using computer tomography and plain radiographs. Their results suggest that this muscle may play an important role in maintaining the posture of the cervical spine. Conley *et al.* (1995) have investigated the magnetic resonance images of cervical spinal muscles. By assessing the exercise-induced contrast shift in T2 signals, the physiological functions of cervical muscles, such as semispinalis capitis and cervicis, splenis capitis, sternocleidomastoid, longus capitis and colli, scalene and levator scapulae, have been validated. Vasavada *et al.* (1998) have employed computer modelling techniques to investigate the effect of muscle morphometry affecting the mechanical moment and range of motion generated by the cervical spinal muscles. Bartons and Hayes (1996) have devised and validated a new method to assess the isometric strength of neck flexor with electromyogram. They have employed this method to compare the neck strength between healthy volunteers and patients with unilateral neck pain and headaches. Statistically significant decreases in the muscle forces have been found in patients with neck pain. These studies have quantified the physiological functions of cervical spinal muscles and the value of studying neck muscle has been explained.

NEUROLOGY OF THE CERVICAL SPINE

Investigation of the neurology of the cervical spine used to be focused either on the spinal cord or spinal nerves. Investigation of the neural tissues embedded in different parts of the cervical spine is, however, rarely reported. McLain (1994) has investigated 21 cervical facet capsules and found that the capsule is innervated by different types of mechanoreceptors, including type I, II, III and nociceptors. He has then proposed that the facet joint capsule is closely monitored by the central nervous system. These results suggest that the neural inputs of these receptors may be crucial for the proprioception and pain sensation of the cervical spine. Disabling this monitoring system may then cause abnormal stress to the cervical spine, leading to mechanical disorders. Swinkles and Dolan (1998) have also investigated the joint sense of the thoracic and lumbar spine, using an electromagnetic motion tracking system. Good repeatability in establishing different postures has been shown. As compared with the thoracic and lumbar spine, it is speculated that a sensitive joint sense is particularly important for the cervical spine. This is because a fast and accurate joint sense is necessary to prevent the head and neck from injuries.

INTERVERTEBRAL DISC

Investigation of intervertebral disc functions is important. This is because a majority of spinal disorders are believed to be associated with the malfunction of the disc. Although it has been generally accepted that the disc can facilitate the motion of the spine, evidence to show that migration of the nucleus pulposus during flexion and extension of the spine has not been reported until recently (Fennell *et al.*, 1996). Using the finite element analysis method, Lu *et al.* (1996) studied the relationship between the disc height and the mechanical functions of the disc. Their results have shown that a variation of the disc height will affect the axial displacement, posterolateral disc bulge and the tensile stress in the peripheral annulus fibres. The importance of the disc height as related to its mechanical functions has been well discussed in this study. Kokubun *et al.* (1996) investigated the vertebral end plate of 20 surgical patients with cervical disc herniation. Cartilaginous end plate type of herniation has been found to be the most common type of disorders and the cleft patterns in the end plate provide useful information to study the degeneration of the cervical disc. Gruber and Hanley (1998) have also investigated the histochemistry and immunohistochemistry of the disc in 33 surgically treated patients. An abnormal apoptosis rate has been found in the disc cells. However, the cause of premature cell death remains unknown. Kang *et al.* (1995) investigated the biochemistry of the herniated cervical disc. Their results suggest that the biochemical substances released during the degeneration of the disc, such as metalloproteinases, nitric oxide, interleukin-6 and prostaglandin E^2 , may be associated with the patho-physiology of radiculopathy.

TRAUMA OF THE CERVICAL SPINE

"Whiplash" injury is probably one of the most common types of cervical spinal injuries in developed countries, due to the popularity of using automobiles. As compared with other cervical spinal injuries, some post-"whiplash" injured patients may be associated with psychological symptoms and/or medicolegal issues (Ratliff, 1997), which can increase the difficulties in identifying the sources of the symptoms. As a result, treatment may be hindered. As persistent neck pain and regular application of sick leave or pension will cause a significant impact on the society, further studies in "whiplash" injury are required.

Grauer *et al.* (1997) and Panjabi *et al.* (1998) have developed a cervical spinal model to investigate the mechanics of the cervical spine. A cadaveric cervical spine is mounted on a cart with a fixed track. The cart is then accelerated with strong springs and collided with a brake, in order to simulate "whiplash" trauma. The alignment of the cervical spine was found to be S-shaped during the impact, which was not reported before. These studies suggest that assessment of the biomechanics of the cervical spine will be helpful in explaining the pathomechanism of the trauma. This will be particularly crucial in planning the treatment for patients with "whiplash" injury.

As a specific lesion of the cervical spine may not be easily identified in most patients, treatment will then be limited. Evaluation of the different types of treatment for patients with "whiplash" injury is therefore necessary. Borchgrenvink *et al.* (1998) compared the treatment outcomes of 201 patients with "whiplash" injuries in Norway, using a randomised control trial study. Treatment outcomes were assessed with different subjective measurements. In a re-assessment six months later, a better outcome was found in patients who were encouraged to participate in their daily activities, as compared with those who were absent from work for long time or who relied on collars to immobilise their neck during the first two weeks after the injury.

DIAGNOSTIC IMAGING

As computer tomography and magnetic resonance imaging (MRI) are non-invasive clinical assessment methods and can provide three-dimensional images of the spine, these techniques provide valuable information, which assists in the diagnosis of cervical spinal disorders. However, these methods do have their own limitations. Extensive studies have been performed to improve the reliability of these diagnostic techniques.

Schellhas *et al.* (1996) have compared the sensitivities of MRI and discography in the assessment of cervical discogenic pain. 10 life long asymptomatic subjects and 10 chronic neck pain patients participated. The intervertebral discs of the cervical spine of these participants were assessed using both MRI and discography. Their results suggests that significant tears in the annulus fibrous of the cervical disc are relatively less easy to detect with MRI, even though MRI is commonly regarded as the golden standard in diagnostic imaging. Therefore, any interpretation of diagnostic images should be made carefully and should be correlated with the clinical findings of patients.

Dynamic assessment of cervical spine images is another new developing research area. Muhle *et al.* (1998) modified the assessment procedures of MRI to investigate the subarachnoid space and spinal cord in 40 healthy subjects. Images of the cervical spine were taken in every 10° intervals, from 50° of flexion to 30° of extension. Changes of the subarachnoid space in relation to the spinal cord were assessed in these studies. This technique is found to be useful to correlate the images and functions of the cervical spine.

TREATMENT OF CERVICAL SPINAL DISORDERS

There is plenty of ongoing research which investigate new treatment techniques or which investigate how to improve the effectiveness and efficiency of the current treatment for cervical spinal disorders. As the resources of healthcare systems are limited and the expectations of treatment outcome in the general population are increasing, medical professionals are frequently required to account for their diagnoses and decisions. Therefore, evaluative studies of treatment cost and effectiveness are encouraged by most funding bodies and this forms the latest trend in cervical spinal disorders research.

For example, Skargen *et al.* (1997) investigated the costs and treatment outcomes of chiropractic and physiotherapy in the management of 323 patients who have either neck or back pain. The patients were randomly assigned to chiropractic and physiotherapy treatment groups. Using different types of self-rating measurement, such as visual analogue pain scale and the Oswestry pain disability questionnaire, the patients' treatment outcomes were reassessed six months after their treatment courses. Results have shown the two types of treatment methods are equally effective in reducing the patients' symptoms. No significant difference in the direct and indirect costs of these treatment has been found. In order to investigate the efficacy of different types of treatment methods for cervical spinal disorders, such as physiotherapy, manipulation, cervical collar and surgery, prospective randomised clinical trials are commonly performed (Persson *et al.*, 1997; Jordan *et al.*, 1998). The results have also suggested that these treatment options are equally effective in the management of patients with cervical spinal disorders.

Although a majority of patients with cervical spinal disorders can be managed with conservative treatment, some patients do not respond well to that. Surgical interventions are then indicated. There is also plenty of ongoing research in studying the surgical treatment for cervical spinal disorders, including investigation of different surgical techniques, long term surgical effects and surgical complications. For examples, Grob *et al.* (1994) have compared the effectiveness of wiring and plating techniques in the fixation of the occipitocervical joints in patients with rheumatoid arthritis. Hilibrand *et al.* (1997) performed a 20-year retrospective study to evaluate the success rate of anterior cervical spinal fusion which is next to a previous arthodesis. Using a multicentre study design, An *et al.* (1995) investigated the effectiveness of allograft with demineralised bone matrix to perform cervical fusion, instead of autogenous bone graft. Lowery and McDonough (1998) investigated the risks and complications of anterior cervical plating. Although rehabilitation of patients with spinal surgery is crucial, little research has been done in post-operative management of patients with spinal surgery. Further studies are therefore required, as an effective rehabilitation programme will be helpful in optimising surgical outcomes and preventing the recurrence of cervical spinal disorders.

EPIDEMIOLOGY

Investigation of the prevalence and incident rates of diseases is useful to identify risk factors related to the occurrence of disease. Preventive measurements can then be made. Also, these data will provide substantial information for both decision making and further studies. Therefore, the value of epidemiological studies of cervical spinal disorders should not be under-estimated. An *et al.* (1994) have investigated the association between cigarette smoking and surgically confirmed herniated disc diseases. Continued smoking has been speculated to aggravate discogenic or radicular symptoms of patients with intervertebral disc disease. Bovim *et al.* (1994) and Barnekow-Bergkvist *et al.* (1998) have investigated the prevalence and symptoms of neck pain in the general population of Norway and Sweden respectively. However, any generalisation of these results to a local society should be done with caution. This is because the validity and reliability of epidemiological data depends on a number of factors, including sample size, cultural background and social values, etc. It is therefore necessary to carry out regular studies to reflect the needs of a specific society. Lau *et al.* (1996) investigated the prevalence and risk factors of neck pain in two housing blocks in Hong Kong. The one-year prevalence rates of neck pain in men and women were found to be 15% and 17% respectively. In contrast to overseas reports, neck pain is relatively common in wealthy population in Hong Kong, rather than the working class.

WORK-RELATED CERVICAL SPINAL DISORDERS

As cervical spinal disorders is a disabling disease, the productivity and efficiency of workers will decrease if they suffer from a neck-shoulder pain. Therefore, special attention must be given to study work-related cervical spinal disorders, particularly in minimising the financial conflicts between employers and employees. Current research in this area is relatively comprehensive, including investigation of risk factors for a particular occupation (Johansson and Rubenowitz, 1994), assessment techniques for the evaluation of work-related cervical spinal disorders (Hagen *et al.*, 1997) and establishment of physical capacity database for comparison (Mayer *et al.* 1994a;b).

The research topics included in this chapter are meant to be an introduction for readers only. The diversity and scale of research in cervical spinal disorders are definitely greater than can be covered in this chapter. Having stated this, readers are encouraged to read up on the latest developments in this field. This will be helpful in improving the success rate in the rehabilitation of patients with cervical spinal disorders.

References:

An H.S., Silveri C.P., Simpson M., File P., Simmons C., Simeone F.A., Balderston R.A. Comparison of smoking habits between patients with surgically confirmed herniated lumbar and cervical disc disease and controls. J Spinal Disord 1994;7:369-73.

An H.S., Simpson J.M., Glover M., Stephany J. Comparison between allograft plus demineralised bone matrix versus autograft in anterior cervical fusion. A prospective multicentre study. Spine 1995;20:2211-6.

Barnekow-Bergkvist M., Hedberg G.E., Janlert U., Jansson E. Determinants of self-reported neck-shoulder and low back symptoms in a general population. Spine 1998;23:235-43.

Barton P.M., Hayes K.C. Neck flexor muscle strength, efficiency, and relaxation times in normal subjects and subjects in unilateral neck pain and headache. Arch Phys Med Rehabil 1996;77:680-7.

Borchgrevink G.E., Kaasa A., McDonagh D., Stiles T.C., Haraldseth O., Lereim I. Acute treatment of whiplash neck sprain injuries. A randomized trial of treatment during the first 14 days after a car accident. Spine 1998;23:25-31.

Bovim G., Schrader H., Sand T. Neck pain in the general population. Spine 1994;19:1307-9.

Conley M.S., Meyer R.A., Bloomberg J.J., Feeback D.L., Dudley G.A. Noninvasive analysis of human neck muscle function. Spine 1995;20:2505-12.

Fennell A.J., Jones A.P., Hukins D.W.L. Migration of the nucleus pulposus within the intervertebral disc during flexion and extension of the spine. Spine 1996;21:2753-7.

Grauer J.N., Panjabi M.M., Cholewicki J., Nibu K., Dvorak J. Whiplash produces an S-shaped curvature of the neck with hyperextension at lower levels. Spine 1997;22:2489-94.

Grob D., Dvorak J., Panjabi M.M., Antinnes J.A. The role of plate and screw fixation in occipitocervical fusion in rheumatoid arthritis. Spine 1994;19:2545-51.

Gruber H.E., Hanley E.N. Analysis of ageing and degeneration of the human intervertebral disc. Comparison of surgical specimens with normal controls. Spine 1998;23:751-7.

Hagen K.B., Harms-Ringdahl K., Enger N.O., Hedenstad R., Morten J. Relationship between subjective neck disorders and cervical spine mobility and motion-related pain in male machine operators. Spine 1997;22:1501-7.

Hilibrand A.S., Yoo J.U., Carlson G.D., Bohlman H.H., The success of anterior cervical arthodesis adjacent to a previous fusion. Spine 1997;22:1574-9.

Johansson J.A., Rubenowitz S. Risk indicators I. The psychosocial and physical work environment for work-related neck, shoulder and low back symptoms: A study among blue- and white-collar workers in eight companies. Scand J Rehab Med 1994;26:131-42.

Jordan A., Bendix T., Nielsen H., Hansen F.R., Høst D., Winkel A. Intensive training, physiotherapy, or manipulation for patients with chronic neck pain. A prospective, single-blinded, randomized clinical trial. Spine 1998;23:311-9.

Kang J.D., Gerogescu H.I., McIntyre-Larkin L., Stefanovic-Racic M., Evans C.H. Herniated cervical intervertebral discs spontaneously produce matrix metalloproteinases, nitric oxide, interleukin-6, and prostaglandin E_2. Spine 1995;20:2373-8.

Kokubun S., Sakurai M., Tanaka Y. Cartilaginous endplate in cervical disc herniation. Spine 1996;21:190-5.

Lau E.M.C., Sham A., Wong K.C. The prevalence of and risk factors for neck pain in Hong Kong Chinese. J Public Health Med 1996;18:396-9.

Lowery G.L., McDonough R.F. The significance of hardware failure in anterior cervical plate fixation. Patients with 2- to 7-year follow-up. Spine 1998;23:181-7.

Lu Y.M., Hutton W.C., Gharpuray V.M. Can variations in intervertebral disc height affect the mechanical function of the disc? Spine 1996;21:2208-17.

Mayer T., Gatchel R.J., Keeley J., Mayer H., Richling D. A male incumbent worker industrial database. Part II: cervical spinal physical capacity. Spine 1994a;19:762-4.

Mayer T., Gatchel R.J., Keeley J., Mayer H., Richling D. A male incumbent worker industrial database. Part III: lumbar/cervical functional testing. Spine 1994b;19:765-70.

Mayoux-Benhamou M.A., Revel M., Vallée C., Roudier R., Barbet J.P., Bargy F. Longus colli has a postural function on cervical curvature. Surg Radiol Anat 1994;16:367-71.

McLain R.F. Mechanoreceptor ending in human cervical facet joints. Spine;1994;495-501.

Muhle C., Wiskirchen J., Weinert D., Falliner A., Wesner F., Brinkmann G., Heller M. Biomechanical aspects of the subarachnoid space and cervical cord in healthy individuals examined with kinematic magnetic resonance imaging. Spine 1998;23:556-67.

Panjabi M.M., Cholewicki J., Nibu K., Babat L.B., Dvorak J. Simulation of whiplash trauma using whole cervical spine specimens. Spine 1998;23:17-24.

Panjabi M.M., Oxland T., Takata K., Goel V., Duranceau J., Krag M. Articular facets of the human spine. Spine 1993;18:1298-310.

Persson L.C.G., Moritz U., Brandt L., Carlsson C.A. Cervical radiculopathy: Pain, muscle weakness and sensory loss in patients with cervical radiculopathy treated with surgery, physiotherapy or cervical collar. A prospective, controlled study. Eur Spine J 1997;6:256-66.

Ratliff A.H.C. Whiplash injuries. J Bone Joint Surg 1997;79B:517-9.

Schellhas K.P., Smith M.D., Gundry C.R., Pollei S.R. Cervical discogenic pain. Prospective correlation of magnetic resonance imaging and discography in asymptomatic subjects and pain sufferers. Spine 1996;21:300-12.

Skargren E.I., Öberg B.E., Carlsson P.G., Gade M. Cost and effectiveness analysis of chiropractic and physiotherapy treatment for low back and neck pain. Six-month follow-up. Spine 1997;2167-77.

Swinkels A., Dolan P. Regional assessment of joint position sense in the spine. Spine 1998;23:590-7.

Vasavada A.N., Li S., Delp S.L. Influence of muscle morphometry and moment arms on the moment-generating capacity of human neck muscles. Spine 1998;23:412-22.

Yoganandan N., Kumaresan S., Voo L., Pintar F.A. Finite element applications in human cervical spine modeling. Spine 1996;21:1824-24.

CHAPTER 19

OUTCOME ASSESSMENT OF NECK PAIN REHABILITATION

Lawrence C.W. Fung

INTRODUCTION

This chapter is aimed at introducing readers to the general concepts and objectives of outcome assessment in the context of contemporary healthcare practices. The importance and needs of outcome assessment are explained in light of the finite healthcare resources and rising public expectation and demand. Particular emphasis is given to the dimensions and types of outcome assessment in conjunction with the complexity of the modern era of healthcare practices. Examples in outcome assessments of neck pain rehabilitation are highlighted and the future development of outcome measures for neck pain rehabilitation is discussed.

WHAT IS OUTCOME ASSESSMENT?

The dictionary definition of outcome is "end-result or effect". To be concerned with outcomes is simply to be concerned with the linkage or causal relationships between antecedent and the resultant effects or events. But in the context of healthcare and services, the meaning of outcome will take on a broader perspective. In addition to the description of end-results as consequences of inputs or processes, it is also defined in terms of the achievement of or failure to achieve desired goals (Wilkin *et al.*, 1992). Subsequent to these broadened dimensions of outcome, the element of assessment or analysis is embraced as an integral part in the context of health outcomes. The definition of outcomes remain debatable, due to the diversity in the types and nature of inputs, processes and end-results to be included in the context of health outcomes. The United Kingdom Clearing House on Health Outcomes had collected a selection of possible definitions taken from a wide

range of sources. Examples of this selection are presented below to illustrate
the differences of focus in varied aspects of health outcomes.

"(The) results of healthcare processes." (Baumberg *et al.*, 1995)

*"Outcome to the individual, essentially comes down to how comfortable, how
accessible and how appropriate will be the care that is offered between the
onset of mortal illness and death."* (Best, 1988)

*"The attributable effect of an intervention or its lack on a previous health
state."* (Great Britain: Department of Health, 1994)

*"Evaluating health outcomes involves determining the effect of the utilization
and provision of health services on the health status of the population. The
major and central question is: What impact do health services have on the
health of the population?"* (Hall *et al.*, 1984)

*"The end results of medical interventions and processes. These can be
assessed in terms of mortality, morbidity, physiological measures and,
increasingly, more subjective patient-based assessments of health."*
(Jenkinson, 1994)

*"A (health status) measure used in the context of assessing the effects of a
(healthcare) intervention, or lack of intervention, or for measuring the extent
to which a desired outcome or end-state is achieved."* (Long, 1996)

*"An outcome is a natural or artificially designed point in the care of an
individual or population suitable for assessing the effect of an intervention, or
lack of intervention, on the natural history of a condition."* (McCallum, 1993)

*"...a change in the health of an individual, group of people or population
which is attributable to an intervention or series of interventions."* (NSW
Health Department, 1992)

*"Outcome is a relative value. It is a measure of change, the end point is
compared with the situation at the start of the study period."* (Pynsent *et al.*,
1993)

*"A health outcome is a result of any health intervention. Health indicators are
measures of outcomes. Outcomes may apply to individuals, populations or
workers."* (Rubin, 1993)

Common to this array of outcome definitions are several key concepts inherent to the assessment of health outcomes. Firstly, there is a wide range of antecedents or interventions upon which outcomes are measured for a single condition. These include various types of clinical treatment and healthcare interventions, as well as different ways and processes of health service provision and utilisation. It is imperative that those outcomes to be assessed are indeed linked to the interventions or the processes of healthcare practices and are not just a different state of health or due to natural recovery. Examples of outcome studies in various types of physiotherapy treatment for neck pain rehabilitation, including clinical trials of mobilisation, manipulation, neck collar, transcutaneous electrical nerve stimulation, massage, as well as heat and cold therapy, can be found in the review written by Hurwitz *et al.* (1996). Evaluation of service provision outcomes can be found in the studies reported by Kamwendo *et al.* (1991) on the effect of neck school in medical secretaries and by Takala *et al.* (1994) on the effect of group gymnastics at workplace.

Secondly, measures of outcome assessment vary, including mortality, morbidity, physiological functions, physical performance, patient satisfaction and quality of life. The choice of outcome measures depends on the intended use or objectives of outcome evaluation (to be discussed in the subsequent section). Examples of outcome measures for neck pain rehabilitation are pain rating and neck motion evaluation (Hagen *et al.*, 1997).

Thirdly, health outcomes are usually measured against pre-determined or desired goal(s). Possible desirable outcomes must be made known to different participants in the healthcare interaction, including patients who receive the medical care, clinicians who provide treatment, managers who monitor the intervention, fund providers who support the health services, and the society which pays for the resources. Given the complexity of today's healthcare services and technologies, it is not uncommon for healthcare to have a multitude of desired goals, which in turn demands a handful of outcome measures for its representation. Therefore, pain ratings and neck motion evaluation alone may not be sufficient to represent the outcomes of neck pain rehabilitation. It is essential to establish new linkages amongst these outcomes, although it would not be surprising to have conflicting outcomes from different participants equipped with different views and expectations towards desirable outcomes. A full restoration of neck motion as targeted by therapists may not be valued much by patients, who strive for a complete cure of pain, although this wish may be considered as unrealistic by therapists.

Fourthly, time scales for assessing the achievement of outcomes must also be defined. An outcome measure provides information in terms of longitudinal assessment of a change in health status from a particular point of time to another, for example, the change in the severity of neck pain over time.

By contrast, a health status measure is a cross-sectional assessment of health status at a particular point in time.

In order to be considered an outcome measure, the instrument must be responsive to changes over time. The time scales for these longitudinal assessments must be specified to show meaningful outcomes achieved by the patient at the individual level and can be standardised to allow comparison at the group level. At the individual level, the common time scale chosen is usually between the initial treatment and discharge of a patient. At the group level, the duration between the first and subsequent assessments (e.g. after eight weeks of treatment) may need to be standardised to compare the treatment outcomes for the particular group of patients in relation to their initial health conditions. Furthermore, the traditional end-point of outcome assessment at the discharge of a patient is being increasingly challenged to include post-discharge outcomes and the patient's overall well-being over the entire course of the disease. Therefore, a neck pain patient may need to follow up for say three to six months after discharge, to assess the effectiveness of treatment on neck pain and mobility.

WHY DO WE NEED OUTCOME ASSESSMENT?

An ex-editor of the New England Journal of Medicine (Relman, 1988) proposed three revolutions in the modern age of medicine in the United States. The first stage was the era of expansion in both medical technologies, financing of medical services and facilities. The second stage was the era of cost containment to stop the escalating growth in healthcare expenditures. The last stage was the era of assessment and accountability in which the focus was directed towards the quality and effectiveness of healthcare. The emphasis was not on blind cost containment, but on a balance between assessment of gains achieved for certain costs and accountability for those costs incurred. In our local scenario, perhaps we are also entering the last stage of assessment for quality and accountability for healthcare practices and effectiveness. With the reality of decreasing healthcare resources and the increase of public expectation and demand for health services, most outcome assessments are targetted to reduce healthcare expenditures and while maintaining high quality patient care.

Although the interest in outcome assessment was stimulated by the need for budget cuts in healthcare expenditure and by the expectation of returning patients quickly to previous functional levels (Lansky *et al.*, 1992), yet other driving forces of outcome assessment cannot be ruled out and they are mainly due to policy and quality concerns. Prompted by unexplained variations in practices, appropriateness of care, effectiveness of treatment and uncertainties of outcomes, Ellwood (1988) proposed that the development of "outcome management" should adopt different ways so as to improve clinical practice and assess medical effectiveness. This signified the beginning of outcome movement in the late 1980s and had important implications for the healthcare practices of today. As a result, a consensus was arrived at regarding the centrality of the patient's viewpoint in defining medical care outcomes and the goal of medical care in achieving the well-being and an effective life for the patient (Ware *et al.*, 1992).

Parallel to these paradigm shifts in focus, from short episodes of illness to long-term follow-up of patients and from provider-defined to patient-perceived outcomes, was the development of measurement instruments incorporating patients as judges of medical outcomes.

In the context of neck pain rehabilitation, outcome assessment enables the identification of the effects of practice variations on outcomes between settings or between therapists, such as those arising from practices of pure manual therapy versus pure physical modalities. The effects of variations in the mode of services, such as quantity and frequency of treatment, and the criteria of discharging patients should be examined, particularly in relation to neck pain reduction and returning to work. Inappropriate practices, such as lack of re-assessment and failure to modify treatment plan according to condition change, may require evidence from outcome assessment for its rectification. Ineffectiveness of treatment, such as electrical nerve stimulation for cervical spondylolisthesis or neck school for mechanical neck disorders, may only be unveiled systematically and quantitatively by outcome assessment.

Uncertainty of outcomes on introduction of new treatment modalities, such as pulsed electromagnetic therapy for acute neck pain may also need to be investigated by outcome assessment for its justification and substantiation (Foley *et al.*, 1990).

From previous discussions, numerous objectives for outcome assessment can be summarised as follows: to reduce cost, to inform priority setting and resource allocation, to increase the accountability of services, to empower patients and involve them in service planning and evaluation, to help set, monitor and improve standards of care, to eliminate poor/unnecessary practice and promote good practice and to evaluate new services.

TYPES OF OUTCOME ASSESSMENT

As mentioned previously, there is a broad range of healthcare activities to be evaluated accompanied with corresponding sets of outcome measurements.

These good mixtures of outcome assessments can be grouped into several categories, representing different perspectives linked with different participants involved in the outcome assessment. There are basically three different groups of participants in an outcome assessment and each group of participants has different perspectives and needs with regard to the outcomes of a healthcare intervention or service. These three types of perspectives represent the perspectives of clinicians, patients and organisations and hence the names of three outcomes: clinical outcomes, patient outcomes and organisational outcomes respectively.

Clinical outcomes

Clinical outcomes represent the perspectives of clinicians or therapists providing care to patients and are mostly concerned with the efficacy of treatment. Traditionally, a treatment is considered to be efficacious if it is successful in saving lives, arresting pathology and curing disease as quickly as possible. In today's healthcare practices, the context of the disease process has been expanded to embrace a hierarchical level of concepts: impairment, disability and handicap. Impairment refers to dysfunction at organ level and is congruent to the limitation of neck mobility, weakening of neck postural muscles and muscles of upper extremity, etc., in cervical spine disorders.

Disability refers to dysfunction at body level and is congruent to difficulties in performing daily living activities, such as reading, writing, carrying heavy objects and recreation activities. Handicap refers to dysfunction at person level and is congruent to the difficulties in assuming one's social role, for example a teacher, clerk or even a housewife, due to neck pain. In the arena of modern healthcare practices, a successful clinical outcome should therefore be able to address those of the impairment outcomes, disability outcomes and handicap outcomes (Whyte, 1994).

Besides, linkages or causal relationships between this hierarchy of impairment, disability and handicap outcomes must be demonstrated before a successful clinical outcome can be achieved. An increase in pain free range of neck movement after a course of manual therapy must be shown to improve a patient's tolerance in keyboard work, which in turn enables him to resume his normal work as a computer operator.

Patient outcomes

Patient outcomes represent the perspectives of patients themselves and are mostly concerned with those things that patients experienced, interpreted, evaluated, reported and valued above all. In effect, these outcomes encompass the subjective feelings and perceptions of patients on the efficacy, effectiveness and benefits of treatment or services measured against their own expectations and well-beings. These patient outcomes extend beyond the disease to other aspects affecting patients' comfort, convenience, satisfaction and ultimately their overall well-beings and quality of life (Rupp *et al.*, 1997). For this reason, patient outcomes may also be termed as humanistic outcomes (Jones *et al.*, 1995).

Therefore, a patient's satisfaction on the types and processes of treatment and services received, such as the ease of access to the service, the amount of waiting time before getting an appointment and the attitude of staff may all be regarded as elements of patient outcomes. Furthermore, a patient's perception on the effects of treatment may be one of the outcome indicators even more important than those clinical outcomes measured by therapist. And it is not uncommon for these patient outcomes to be different from clinical outcomes due to differences in perspectives. So a complete reversal of signs in objective findings (including a full range of neck movement and a non-tender cervical spine) might be regarded as successful clinical outcomes by the therapist, yet may not be valued as much by the patient who complained of symptoms only on carrying heavy objects.

Recently, these patient outcomes have become important indicators for service prioritisation and resource allocation in light of the pressure of public accountability and the advocate for quality patient-centered care. Although there is consensus of the importance of assessing these humanistic aspects of care, yet there is no agreement regarding standardising their measurement techniques. Nowadays, these humanistic outcomes are mostly measured through patient questionnaires, especially for those instruments measuring patients' quality of life. These health-related quality-of-life measures, HRQoL, may be generic (measuring aspects of HRQoL that may be applicable to a variety of patients with different conditions) or disease-specific (measuring aspects of HRQoL that are specific to patients with a particular disease or condition).

Organisational outcomes

Organisational outcomes represent the perspective of the organisation which includes the department rendering the service, the hospital as the overall healthcare provider and even the society utilising and monitoring the services at large. Areas of major concern from these various parties are summarised as economic, quality and management outcomes. Economic outcomes are undoubtedly the most important consideration from organisational perspective.

Healthcare is now confronting the reality that even as medical care becomes more sophisticated, the ability or willingness of society to pay for this care is reaching an end. What was once a maxim, "the best care that medicine can provide" is slowly being replaced by a new slogan, "the best care we can afford". This has forced the institution to confront the idea of providing the best possible care within available resources. As resources are increasingly scarce, economisation of healthcare is driving the current trend towards embracing economic outcomes in healthcare practices and management.

Common examples of economic outcome studies include those of cost-effectiveness studies, cost-benefit analysis and cost-utility analysis. It is through these studies that decision can be made comparing the expected gain of intervention against the expected cost of that intervention. Accurate calculation of the expected intervention cost in the first place, therefore, becomes crucial to maximise the economic outcomes of intervention.

Examples of these costs in neck pain rehabilitation in an out-patient department include the duration of each treatment session, the amount of treatment modalities offered and the number of treatment sessions required for discharging a patient. Sometimes, this cost consideration may extend to include those of the patient costs, such as taking the working day off to attend treatment and the amount of money spent on home therapy appliance, such as TENS machine.

Quality and management outcomes are more the concern of department and hospital managers and are usually measured on an aggregation basis, instead of an individual basis. Examples of quality outcomes include mortality and morbidity rate, complication rate, recurrence rate and the number of patient complaints. Examples of management outcomes include health services utilisation, patient turnover rate, waiting time and number of patients in waiting list.

From the above discussion, it is well demonstrated that outcomes for a healthcare intervention are complex, multi-dimensional and inter-related. The choice of outcome assessment depends largely on its intended use and objectives. It is not uncommon for a multitude of outcomes to represent the efficacy and effectiveness of an intervention. There are no fixed rules in selecting appropriate outcome measures for a particular purpose. However, a common rule-of-thumb is to employ clinical outcomes for treatment efficacy study and to include patient and organisational outcomes for treatment effectiveness study.

CRITERIA OF OUTCOME MEASURES

In order for outcome assessment to accurately evaluate clinical practices, inform service planning and monitoring, prioritise resource allocation and reduce costs, instruments for measuring and reporting results of outcome assessment ~ commonly termed as outcome measures - must be established. To perform specified functions, these outcome measures must satisfy certain basic qualifying criteria. The following are some of the suggestions given by the United Kingdom Clearing House on Health Outcomes.

User centredness

The user centredness of an outcome measure refers to the extent to which it faithfully captures both the content of users' views and the ways in which those views are expressed by users. It is a form of content validity since a measure which aims to capture users' views but does not do so cannot be described as valid. Therefore, a measure capturing the impairment outcomes of neck pain rehabilitation cannot be regarded as valid if the user of the measure is a hospital executive who is only interested in service planning of neck pain rehabilitation.

Psychometrics

In order to be used within routine clinical practice, the measure must be psychometrically sound. Key psychometric properties include: reliability (does the instrument consistently measure the same thing), validity (does the instrument measure what it purports to measure) and responsiveness to change (does the instrument detect changes in health status that are meaningful to the users).

Feasibility

A central issue of concern to users is how practical the measure is for use in routine clinical practice. A majority of outcome measures have been developed within research settings where maximising psychometric properties have led to instruments that require too long a period for use in routine practice.

Other factors such as the length of a questionnaire, its mode of administration and the ease with which it can be scored, interpreted and fed back within clinical settings are as critical to the adoption of measures within routine practice. At the same time, short instruments are in general more likely to be less reliable. Thus, in considering outcome measures appropriate for use within routine practice, a balance is often required between their psychometric properties and their feasibility for use in routine practice.

Finally, limits of patient's ability might also limit the feasibility of outcome measures to be used for a particular group of patients. It has been found that elderly patients had perceptual problems in scoring in the visual analogue scale or numeric rating scale of pain assessment, and self-administered questionnaires may be inappropriate for illiterate patients.

Utility

For a measure to be incorporated as routine practice, it must have clinical and user utility, providing information of the process of decision making. In addition, the measure must be appropriate for the setting where the clinician wishes to use it. Many outcome measures have only been validated for use in particular settings or with specific user populations. It is essential that the validity of a measure, in particular its content validity should be checked before it is used in different settings or with a group of users different from those for which the measure was originally designed.

Quantifiable

A fundamental but not a pre-requisite requirement is for scoring of outcome measures to be quantified in terms of either interval or ordinal scales and which should undergo proper psychometric evaluations. Therefore, an improvement in neck mobility should be reported in terms of degree of motion (as measured by a goniometer or inclinometer) instead of just a qualitative description of the estimated range of mobility.

Examples of outcome measures for neck pain rehabilitation

Examples of outcome measures reported in the literature discussing neck pain rehabilitation or other cervical spine disorders are rather limited and are mainly focused on impairment outcomes. Pain and neck mobility are the two common outcome measures employed by most studies in this area. The visual analogue scale or McGill Pain Questionnaire is often chosen to measure the outcome of pain relief (Schofferman *et al.*, 1994; Hurwitz *et al.*, 1996; Rogers, 1997). Goniometric evaluation is common employed to measure the gain in neck motion (Cassidy *et al.*, 1992; Cassidy *et al.*, 1992; Osterbauer *et al.*, 1992).

Literature reporting the inclusion of disability and patient outcomes has been scarce. This is most likely due to the limitations of these outcome measures in terms of their limited clinical utility for a particular group of patients and their unfeasibility requiring a lengthy administration. For example, Leak *et al.* (1994) reported the use of the Northwick Park Neck Pain Questionnaire to assess a group of rheumatology patients; Vernon & Mior (1991) modified the Oswestry Low Back Pain Index into the Neck Disability Index for the assessment of patients with neck pain; Lavin *et al.* (1997) included the Sickness Impact Profile as the quality of life index as one of the outcome measures. Aker *et al.* (1997) suggested quite a comprehensive range of outcome measures for mechanical neck disorders in their protocol review for the Cochrane Collaboration. Their suggestions, together with the author's are listed in Table 1 to 4 for readers' reference.

Table 1. Measures for impairment outcomes.

pain	visual analogue scale, numeric rating scale, borg scale, McGill Pain Questionnaire, pain drawing.
range of motion	cervical goniometry, inclinometry, tape measure.

Table 2. Measures for disability outcomes.

Neck Disability Index

Northwick Park Neck Pain Questionnaire
(for rheumatology patients).

Beck Depression Inventory
(screening for depression for chronic neck pain patients)

Table 3. Measures for patient outcomes.

Short-Form 36 (SF-36), Sickness Impact Profile.
Hong Kong version of World Health Organization Quality of Life Questionnaire (WHOQOL)
Patient Satisfaction Survey

Table 4. Measures for economic outcomes.

Amount of medication consumed
Number of days for return to work
Number of days off work
Number of sick leave days

FUTURE DEVELOPMENT OF OUTCOME ASSESSMENT

In the modern complexity of healthcare practices, multiple outcomes are often required to address the effectiveness and efficacy of a healthcare intervention. However, development of outcome measures for neck pain and other cervical spine disorders were mainly limited to those of impairment outcomes. Outcome measures specific to cervical disability and quality of life have been lacking so far. The situation is equally bad in the development of local instruments appropriate for the Chinese culture. Problems would still exist even after the development of local instruments if there is no consensus on standardisation of the outcome measures used (in light of multitude of instruments available for the same purpose). Collection of local normative data will only be meaningful after outcome measures have been standardised on a territory-wide basis. These normative outcome data will then possess evaluative, comparative and predictive values on clinical practices between different settings and institutions. It is hoped that future research efforts (outcome research) could be directed towards this outcome movement, which signifies a paradigm shift in our healthcare practices with a more holistic and humanistic outlook (Jette, 1995).

Acknowledgement

Acknowledgement is given to the United Kingdom Clearing House on Health Outcomes for reproduction made for part of the materials contained in the information sheets on health outcomes.

References:

Aker P.D., Gross A.R., Goldsmith C.H., Peloso P. Conservative management of mechanical neck disorders. Part one: manual therapy [Protocol]. In: Bombardier C, Nachemson A, Deyo R, deBie R, Bouter L, Shekelle P, Waddell G, Roland M Guillemin F eds, Back Review Module of The Cochrane Database of Systematic Reviews. The Cochrane Collaboration; Issue 4. Oxford: Update Software 1997.

Baumberg L., Long A., Jefferson J. International workshop: culture and outcomes: Barcelona, Leeds, European Clearing Houses on Health Outcomes, 9-10 June 1995.

Best J. The matter of outcome. Med J Aust 1988;148:651.

Cassidy J.D., Lopes A.A., Yong-Hing K. The immediate effect of manipulation versus mobilization on pain and range of motion in the cervical spine: a randomized controlled trial. J Manip Physiol Ther 1992;15:570-5.

Cassidy J.D., Quon J.A., LaFrance L.J., Yong-Hing K. The effect of manipulation on pain and range of motion in the cervical spine: a pilot study. J Manip Physiol Ther 1992;15:495-500.

Ellwood P.M. Shattuck Lecture – Outcome management. A technology of patient experience. N Eng J Med 1988;318:1549-56.

Foley N.D., Barry C., Coughlan R.J., O'Connor P., Roden D. Pulsed high frequency (27MHz) electromagnetic therapy for persistent neck pain. A double blind, placebo-controlled study of 20 patients. Orthopedics 1990;13:445-51.

Hurwitz E.L., Aker P.D., Adams A.H., Meeker W.C., Shekelle P.G. Manipulation and mobilization of the cervical spine. A systematic review of the literature. Spine 1996;21:1746-59.

Jenkinson C. Measuring health and medical outcomes. London, University College London Press 1994.

Jette A.M. Outcomes Research: Shifting the Dominant Research Paradigm in Physical Therapy. Phys Ther 1995;75:965-70.

Jones A.J., Sanchez L.A. Pharmacoeconomic Evaluation: Applications in Managed Health Care Formulary Decision-Making. Drug Benefit Trends 1995;7:12-34.

Kamwendo K., Linton S.J. A controlled study of the effect of neck school in medical secretaries. Scand J Rehabil Med 1991;23:143-52.

Lansky D., Butler J.B.V., Waller F.T. Using Health Status Measures in the Hospital Setting: From Acute Care to Outcomes Management. Med Care 1992;30:MS57-73.

Lavin R.A., Pappagallo M., Kuhlemeier K.V. Cervical pain: A comparison of three pillows. Arch Phys Med Rehabil 1997;78:193-8.

Leak A.M., Cooper J., Dyer S., Williams K.A., Turner-Stokes L., Frank A.O. The Northwick Park Neck Pain Questionnaire, devised to measure neck pain and disability. Br J Rheumatol 1994;33:469-74.

Long A.F. Outcomes with audit: a process and outcome perspective. Outcomes Briefing 1996;7:5.

McCallum J. What is an outcome and why look at them? Critical Public Health, 1993;4:4.

NSW Health Department. The NSW Health Outcomes Program. New South Wales Public Health Bulletin, 1992;3:135.

Osterbauer P.J., Derickson K.L., Peles J.D., DeBoer K.F., Fuhr A.W., Winters J.M. Three-dimensional head kinematics and clinical outcome of patients with neck injury treated with spinal manipulative therapy: A pilot study. J Manip Physiol Ther 1992;15:501-11.

Pynsent P., Fairbank J., Carr A. Outcome measures in orthopaedics. Oxford, Butterworth Heinemann 1993.

Relman A. Assessment and accountability: the third revolution in medical care. N Engl J Med 1988;319:1220-2.

Rogers R.G. The effects of spinal manipulation on cervical kinesthesia in patients with chronic neck pain: A pilot study. J Manip Physiol Ther 1997;20:80-5.

Rubin G. The NSW Health Outcomes Program. NSW: Health Customer Focus Conference, Wesley Centre 1993:1.

Rupp M.T., Kreling D.H. The impact of pharmaceutical care on patient outcomes: What do we know? Drug Benefit Trends 1997;9:35-47.

Schofferman J., Wasserman S. Successful treatment of low back pain and neck pain after a motor vehicle accident despite litigation. Spine 1994;19:1007-10.

Suggested readings list:

Cole B., Basmajian J. Physical rehabilitation outcome measures. Toronto, Canadian Physiotherapy Association 1994.

Hopkins A., Costain D. Measuring the outcomes of medical care. London, Royal College of Physicians and the King's Fund Centre for Health Services Development, 1990.

Macfarlane R., Hardy D.G. Outcome after head, neck and spinal trauma: a medicolegal guide. Oxford, Butterworth-Heinemann 1997.

Pynsent P.B., Fairbank J.C.T., Carr A. Outcome measures in orthopaedics. Oxford, Butterworth-Heinemann 1993.

Sederer L.I., Dickey B. Outcomes assessment in clinical practice. Baltimore, Williams & Wilkins 1996.

Smith P. Measuring outcome in the public sector. London, Taylor & Francis 1996.